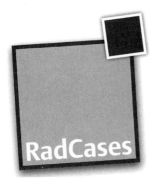

Thoracic Imaging

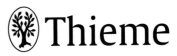

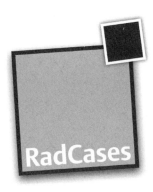

Thoracic Imaging

Edited by

Carlos Santiago Restrepo, MD
Professor of Radiology
Chief of Chest Radiology
University of Texas Health Science Center at San Antonio
San Antonio, Texas

Steven M. Zangan, MD
Assistant Professor of Radiology
University of Chicago Medical Center
Chicago, Illinois

Series Editors

Jonathan Lorenz, MD
Associate Professor of Radiology
Department of Radiology
The University of Chicago
Chicago, Illinois

Hector Ferral, MD
Professor of Radiology
Section Chief, Interventional Radiology
RUSH University Medical Center, Chicago
Chicago, Illinois

Thieme
New York • Stuttgart

Thieme Medical Publishers, Inc.
333 Seventh Ave.
New York, NY 10001

Executive Editor: Timothy Hiscock
Editorial Assistant: Adriana di Giorgio
Editorial Director: Michael Wachinger
Production Editor: Katy Whipple, Maryland Composition
International Production Director: Andreas Schabert
Vice President, International Marketing and Sales: Cornelia Schulze
Chief Financial Officer: James W. Mitos
President: Brian D. Scanlan
Compositor: MPS Content Services
Printer: Sheridan Press

Library of Congress Cataloging-in-Publication Data

Thoracic imaging / edited by Carlos Santiago Restrepo, Steven M. Zangan.
       p. ; cm.—(RadCases)
    Includes bibliographical references.
    ISBN 978-1-60406-187-1
  1. Chest—Radiography—Case studies. I. Restrepo, Carlos Santiago. II. Zangan, Steven M.
III. Series: RadCases.
    [DNLM: 1. Radiography, Thoracic—methods—Case Reports. 2. Diagnosis,
Differential—Case Reports. 3. Tomography, Emission-Computed—methods—Case
Reports. WF 975]
    RC941.T46 2010
    617.5'407572—dc22

                                                                              2010028184

Important note: Medical knowledge is ever-changing. As new research and clinical experience broaden our knowledge, changes in treatment and drug therapy may be required. The authors and editors of the material herein have consulted sources believed to be reliable in their efforts to provide information that is complete and in accord with the standards accepted at the time of publication. However, in view of the possibility of human error by the authors, editors, or publisher of the work herein or changes in medical knowledge, neither the authors, editors, nor publisher, nor any other party who has been involved in the preparation of this work, warrants that the information contained herein is in every respect accurate or complete, and they are not responsible for any errors or omissions or for the results obtained from use of such information. Readers are encouraged to confirm the information contained herein with other sources. For example, readers are advised to check the product information sheet included in the package of each drug they plan to administer to be certain that the information contained in this publication is accurate and that changes have not been made in the recommended dose or in the contraindications for administration. This recommendation is of particular importance in connection with new or infrequently used drugs.

Some of the product names, patents, and registered designs referred to in this book are in fact registered trademarks or proprietary names even though specific reference to this fact is not always made in the text. Therefore, the appearance of a name without designation as proprietary is not to be construed as a representation by the publisher that it is in the public domain.

Printed in the United States

978-1-60406-187-1

To the many teachers who have inspired me in the past.
To the students who inspire me today.
To all those patients who challenge me every day.
—*Carlos Santiago Restrepo*

To Tracie, Max, and Vince.
—*Steven M. Zangan*

RadCases Series Preface

The ability to assimilate detailed information across the entire spectrum of radiology is the Holy Grail sought by those preparing for the American Board of Radiology examination. As enthusiastic partners in the Thieme RadCases Series who formerly took the examination, we understand the exhaustion and frustration shared by residents and the families of residents engaged in this quest. It has been our observation that despite ongoing efforts to improve Web-based interactive databases, residents still find themselves searching for material they can review while preparing for the radiology board examinations and remain frustrated by the fact that only a few printed guidebooks are available, which are limited in both format and image quality. Perhaps their greatest source of frustration is the inability to easily locate groups of cases across all subspecialties of radiology that are organized and tailored for their immediate study needs. Imagine being able to immediately access groups of high-quality cases to arrange study sessions, quickly extract and master information, and prepare for theme-based radiology conferences. Our goal in creating the RadCases Series was to combine the popularity and portability of printed books with the adaptability, exceptional quality, and interactive features of an electronic case-based format.

The intent of the printed book is to encourage repeated priming in the use of critical information by providing a portable group of exceptional core cases that the resident can master. The best way to determine the format for these cases was to ask residents from around the country to weigh in. Overwhelmingly, the residents said that they would prefer a concise, point-by-point presentation of the Essential Facts of each case in an easy-to-read, bulleted format. This approach is easy on exhausted eyes and provides a quick review of Pearls and Pitfalls as information is absorbed during repeated study sessions. We worked hard to choose cases that could be presented well in this format, recognizing the limitations inherent in reproducing high-quality images in print. Unlike the authors of other case-based radiology review books, we removed the guesswork by providing clear annotations and descriptions for all images. In our opinion, there is nothing worse than being unable to locate a subtle finding on a poorly reproduced image even after one knows the final diagnosis.

The electronic cases expand on the printed book and provide a comprehensive review of the entire subspecialty. Thousands of cases are strategically designed to increase the resident's knowledge by providing exposure to additional case examples—from basic to advanced—and by exploring "Aunt Minnie's," unusual diagnoses, and variability within a single diagnosis. The search engine gives the resident a fighting chance to find the Holy Grail by creating individualized, daily study lists that are not limited by factors such as a radiology subsection. For example, tailor today's study list to cases involving tuberculosis and include cases in every subspecialty and every system of the body. Or study only thoracic cases, including those with links to cardiology, nuclear medicine, and pediatrics. Or study only musculoskeletal cases. The choice is yours.

As enthusiastic partners in this project, we started small and, with the encouragement, talent, and guidance of Tim Hiscock at Thieme, continued to raise the bar in our effort to assist residents in tackling the daunting task of assimilating massive amounts of information. We are passionate about continuing this journey, hoping to expand the cases in our electronic series, adapt cases based on direct feedback from residents, and increase the features intended for board review and self-assessment. As the American Board of Radiology converts its certifying examinations to an electronic format, our series will be the one best suited to meet the needs of the next generation of overworked and exhausted residents in radiology.

Jonathan Lorenz, MD
Hector Ferral, MD
Chicago, IL

Preface

Thoracic imaging, from conventional radiographs to more complex modalities, comprises a significant portion of the workload in contemporary radiology departments. Proper observation, analysis, and interpretation of these exams requires thorough understanding of the pathophysiology and imaging manifestations of a broad range of disease processes. In this review of 100 printed and 150 electronic cases, the essential imaging details of a myriad of conditions, both common and uncommon, are presented. We hope this concise review of imaging findings, differential diagnoses, essential facts, and pearls prepares you not only for the board examination, but most importantly, for a lifelong career in radiology.

Acknowledgments

I would like to thank Santiago Martinez, MD (Kansas City, MO), Nelson Luraguiz, MD (Shreveport, LA), Santiago Rossi, MD (Buenos Aires, Argentina), Jorge Carrillo, MD, and Ramon Reina, MD (Bogota, Columbia) for their valuable contributions.

—*Carlos Santiago Restrepo*

I would like to thank Drs. Heber MacMahon and Steven Montner for kindly sharing their voluminous teaching files and offering some of the pearls that have made their way into this review.

—*Steven M. Zangan*

Case 1

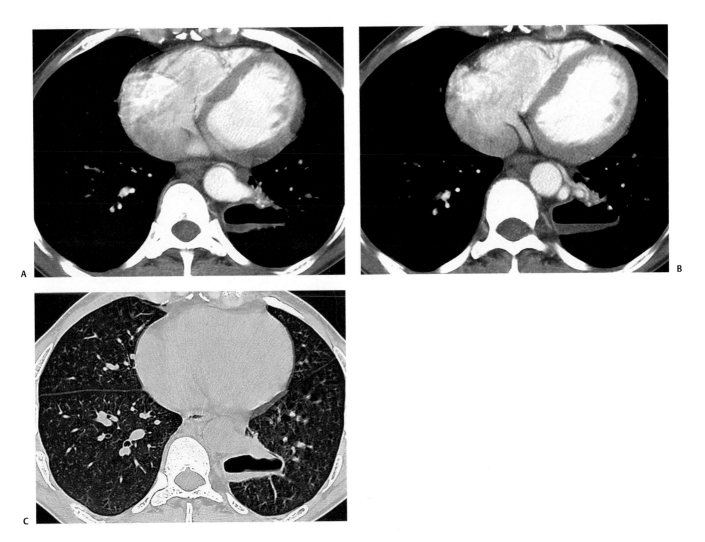

▪ Clinical Presentation

A 23-year-old man with recurrent pneumonia.

■ Imaging Findings

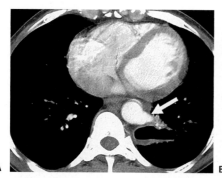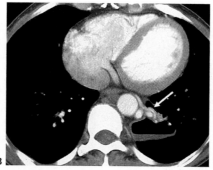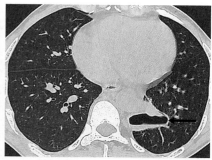

(A–C) Contrast-enhanced thoracic computed tomography. Mediastinal window (A,B) and lung window (C) images demonstrate a well-defined cavitary lesion in the left lower lobe (*black arrow*, C) and an abnormal vessel arising from the lateral aspect of the distal descending thoracic aorta (*white arrow*, A), adjacent to the cavitary lesion. An abnormal vein anterior to the aorta is also present (*white arrow*, B).

■ Differential Diagnosis

- **Pulmonary sequestration (PS):** A parenchymal mass or cavitary lesion in a lower lobe with systemic arterial supply and systemic venous drainage is characteristic of a PS.
- *Lung abscess:* A lung abscess in a lower lobe can present with an appearance similar to that of a PS. Key elements for differentiating between these conditions are the vascular supply and drainage of the abnormality. A pulmonary abscess in a previously normal lung should have a normal pulmonary supply and normal venous return.
- *Intrapulmonary bronchogenic cyst:* A bronchogenic cyst, when located in the pulmonary parenchyma, can also resemble a PS. Again, the vasculature helps in distinguishing between these abnormalities.

■ Essential Facts

- PS is an anomaly of tracheobronchial branching, with an abnormal bronchial connection or obstruction and abnormal systemic arterial supply to the affected lung.
- Common clinical presentations include pneumonia, recurrent infection, cough, and hemoptysis.
- Bronchiectasis, atelectasis, air-fluid levels, and emphysema in the sequestered lung are common.
- Classically, PS has been divided into two major categories: intralobar and extralobar.
- Intralobar sequestration is the most common type (75%), may affect either lower lobe, is likely congenital, and is surrounded by visceral pleura.

- Some cases of intralobar sequestration are probably acquired as a consequence of bronchial obstruction and receive arterial supply from the descending aorta.
- Extralobar sequestration is likely congenital, is seen predominantly in males, and commonly presents relatively early in life. The vast majority of extralobar sequestrations are located in the left lower lobe (90%).
- An extralobar sequestration receives its arterial supply from either the thoracic or the abdominal aorta.
- A large number of extralobar sequestrations are associated with other abnormalities, such as left posterior diaphragmatic hernia (80%), congenital heart disease, and congenital cystic adenomatoid malformation, or they may be connected to the gastrointestinal tract (esophagus or stomach).

✓ Pearls & ✗ Pitfalls

- ✓ Intralobar sequestrations have venous drainage through the pulmonary venous system, whereas extralobar sequestrations have systemic venous drainage through the azygos vein, hemiazygos system, or inferior vena cava.
- ✗ On conventional radiographs, PS can have a wide spectrum of imaging findings, including a solid mass, a cystic lesion, and an air-fluid level, which can be confused with pneumonia, abscess, cyst, and tumor.

Case 2

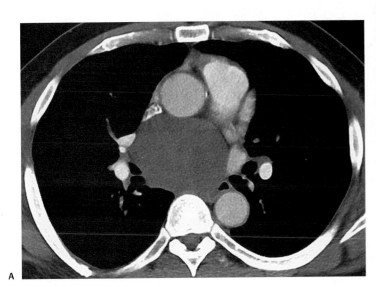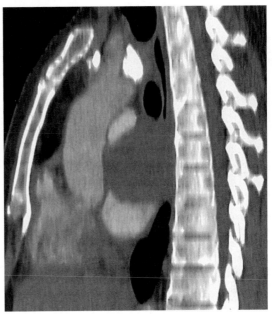

A

B

■ Clinical Presentation

A 52-year-old man with cough and dysphagia and abnormal findings on chest radiograph.

■ Imaging Findings

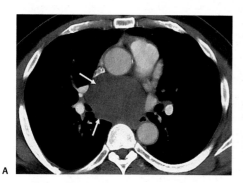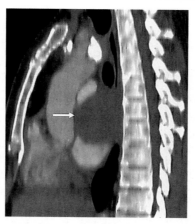

(A,B) Contrast-enhanced thoracic computed tomography (CT). Axial (A) and sagittal (B) re-formations demonstrate a low-density mass with a cystic appearance in the subcarinal region (*arrows*, A) that has a mild mass effect on the esophagus, which is seen between the aorta and the cystic mass (*arrow*, B).

■ Differential Diagnosis

- **Bronchogenic cyst (BC):** An entirely cystic mass adjacent to the trachea or in the subcarinal region is a characteristic presentation of BC.
- *Esophageal (enteric) duplication cyst:* The presentation of an esophageal duplication cyst can be similar or even identical presentation to that of a BC. Esophageal duplication cysts are usually adjacent to or within the esophageal wall.
- *Pericardial cyst:* The most common location of a pericardial cyst is in the cardiophrenic angles, more commonly on the right side.

■ Essential Facts

- BCs are the most common cystic mass of the mediastinum.
- These congenital anomalies result from abnormal ventral budding or branching of the tracheobronchial tree during embryologic development.
- They are lined by respiratory epithelium, and their walls usually contain cartilage and smooth muscle.
- BCs may contain clear serous or dense mucoid material.
- A common location is in the subcarinal region or adjacent to the tracheal wall.
- Other, less common locations include the lung parenchyma and lower neck.
- On CT, a BC appears as a unilocular, smooth, homogeneous, low-density round or oval mass with an imperceptible wall.
- Calcification may develop in the wall of a BC.
- Infection may occur (20% of cases), is more common in intraparenchymal cysts, and is related to communication with the tracheobronchial tree.

■ Other Imaging Findings

- On T2-weighted magnetic resonance sequences, BCs have a high signal intensity. The signal intensity on T1-weighted images is variable, depending on the presence of mucus, protein, or hemorrhage within the cyst.

✓ Pearls & ✗ Pitfalls

- ✓ The majority of BCs are asymptomatic, but occasionally they present with symptoms related to the extrinsic compression of adjacent structures, such as airways or the esophagus.
- ✗ BCs may develop within the lung parenchyma, mimicking lung abscess or malignancy.

Case 3

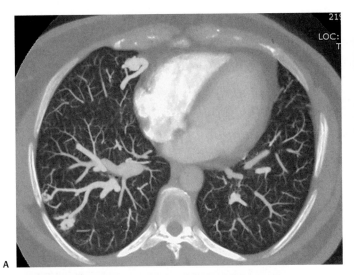

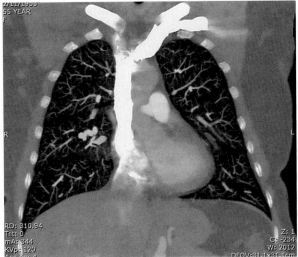

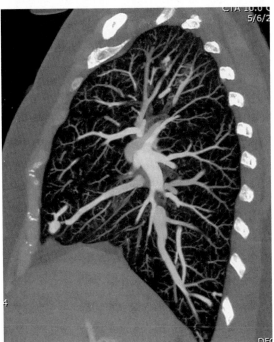

▪ Clinical Presentation

A 55-year-old woman with a history of epistaxis and headache.

■ Imaging Findings

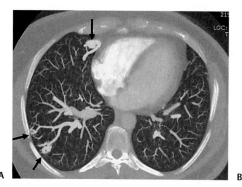 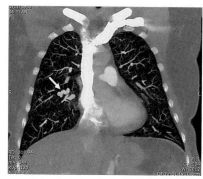 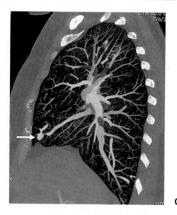

(A–C) Contrast-enhanced computed tomography (CT) of the chest. Axial (A), coronal (B), and sagittal (C) maximum-intensity-projection reconstructions demonstrate multiple dilated vascular structures with prominent connecting vessels throughout the right lung, consistent with arteriovenous (AV) malformations (*arrows*).

■ Differential Diagnosis

- *Hereditary hemorrhagic telangiectasia (HHT; Osler-Weber-Rendu disease):* The clinical triad of telangiectasia, recurrent epistaxis, and multiple-organ AV malformations, in addition to a positive family history with an affected first-degree relative, is characteristic of this condition.
- *Posttraumatic AV fistula:* Trauma can create abnormal fistulous communications between pulmonary arteries and veins. They are usually solitary—not multiple or bilateral, as is often the case in Osler-Weber-Rendu disease.
- *Pulmonary varix:* A pulmonary varix is an abnormal dilatation of a pulmonary vein without AV communication.

■ Essential Facts

- This condition was originally named after Sir William Osler, Frederick Parks Weber, and Henri Rendu.
- HHT is inherited as an autosomal-dominant disorder of variable penetrance (chromosomes 9 and 12).
- It has no gender preference.
- The prevalence is about 1 to 2 per 100,000 persons.
- Abnormal blood vessels affect the skin and mucosa and are also found in the lungs, liver, and central nervous system (CNS).
- Telangiectases are typically small (< 5 mm).
- Recurrent epistaxis (50–80%) is a common clinical presentation.
- Twenty percent of patients affected with HHT have at least one AV malformation in their lungs. In one-third to one-half, the malformations are multiple or bilateral.

- Sixty percent of persons with pulmonary AV malformations have HHT.
- CNS manifestations are seen in 10% of patients, including stroke and brain abscess.
- Strokes in HHT can be hemorrhagic, due to a bleeding AV malformation, or ischemic, due to a paradoxical embolism from a pulmonary AV malformation.

■ Other Imaging Findings

- Color Doppler ultrasound, contrast-enhanced CT, and magnetic resonance imaging are useful modalities for demonstrating hepatic AV malformations in patients with HHT.

✓ Pearls & ✗ Pitfalls

- ✓ When pulmonary AV malformations are large enough to create a significant right-to-left shunt, patients may present with hypoxemia, cyanosis, clubbing, and polycythemia.
- ✗ Pulmonary varices are localized abnormal dilatations of pulmonary veins with no abnormal AV communication and no shunt. They may be congenital or secondary to long-standing pulmonary hypertension, partial anomalous pulmonary venous return, or mitral regurgitation.

Case 4

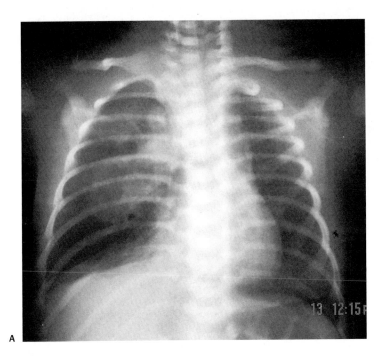

A

Clinical Presentation

A 3-week-old infant with respiratory distress and decreased breath sounds in the right hemithorax.

Further Work-up

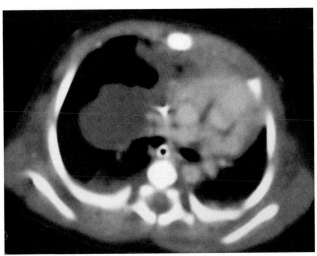

B

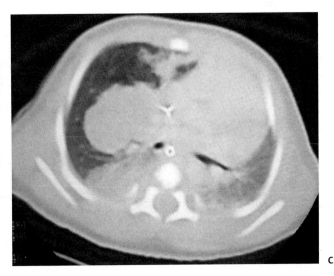

C

◼ Imaging Findings

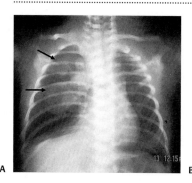 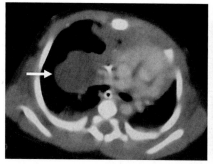 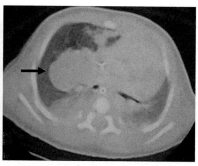

(A) Conventional radiograph shows a well-defined lobulated mass in the right middle and upper lung zones (*arrows*). (B,C) Computed tomography with mediastinal and lung windows confirms the presence of the low-density mass (*arrows*) and atelectasis of the right lower and middle lobes.

◼ Differential Diagnosis

- ***Congenital cystic adenomatoid malformation (CCAM) of the lung:*** In a newborn or a young infant, CCAM of the lung may present as a cyst or mass with a variable degree of compression and mass effect on the adjacent lung and mediastinum.
- *Bronchogenic cyst:* Bronchogenic cyst may also manifest early in infancy, and the presentation may include either a mediastinal or a pulmonary mass or cyst.
- *Lymphangioma/cystic hygroma:* This usually involves the neck and thoracic inlet. Mediastinal involvement can be seen as a cystic lesion.

◼ Essential Facts

- CCAM results from an adenomatous overgrowth of the terminal bronchioles and consequent reduced alveolar growth during abnormal embryogenesis of the bronchoalveolar tissue early in the first trimester.
- This anomalous development of terminal respiratory structures results in the formation of dysplastic tissue, with various communicating cysts lined by adenomatoid respiratory epithelium.
- The abnormally developed lung parenchyma has a relative scarcity of cartilage and an increased amount of elastic tissue.
- The abnormality is more commonly localized to a single lobe, with no lobar preference.
- Prenatal sonographic diagnosis of CCAM is now relatively common, allowing early diagnosis, prenatal counseling, birth planning, and, when required, fetal intervention.
- When large enough, the lesion may compress the esophagus and cause polyhydramnios, or it may compress the ipsilateral lung and produce pulmonary hypoplasia.
- More than half of affected children present with respiratory distress in the neonatal period.
- Malignant transformation into several types of tumors, including rhabdomyosarcoma, bronchoalveolar carcinoma, and pleuropulmonary blastoma, has been reported.
- Treatment is surgical resection.

◼ Other Imaging Findings

- Antenatal magnetic resonance imaging for congenital pulmonary abnormalities has also been reported, but the exact role of this technology has not been completely defined. Some authors have suggested that it may be useful to evaluate any pulmonary hypoplasia and to help predict outcome in fetuses with CCAM.

✓ Pearls & ✗ Pitfalls

- ✓ The most widely used classification is the one developed by Stocker et al., in which lesions are divided into three types, depending on the size of the cyst and histologic criteria:
  - In type 1, one or more cysts more than 2 cm in diameter are surrounded by smaller cysts. The cysts are lined by ciliated columnar epithelium, and their walls are rich in elastic tissue. This is the most common type (50–70%).
  - In type 2 (< 40% of cases), the cysts are less than 2 cm in diameter and lined with cuboidal or columnar epithelium, resembling dilated bronchioles. Type 2 has more commonly been associated with other congenital anomalies, like renal, cardiac, and other pulmonary malformations.
  - In type 3 (10% of cases), the cysts are usually smaller than 0.5 cm in diameter and lined by cuboidal epithelium. This type may appear solid on imaging and gross examination (10%). Type 3 has the worst prognosis.
- ✗ The antenatal diagnosis of congenital lung lesions can be difficult, and several of them can be associated with polyhydramnios. A unilateral intrathoracic echogenic lesion can be due to CCAM or congenital diaphragmatic hernia. Demonstration of the normally positioned stomach and visualization of the diaphragm favors the possibility of CCAM.

Case 5

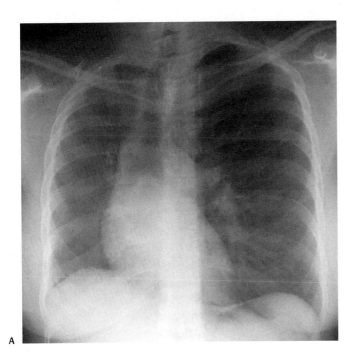

A

Clinical Presentation

A 22-year-old woman with cough and dyspnea.

Further Work-up

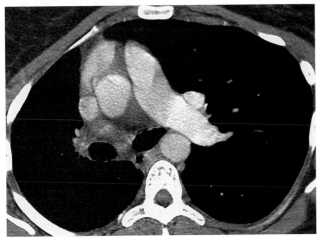

B

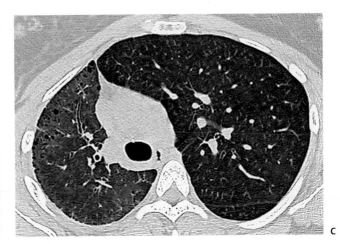

C

■ Imaging Findings

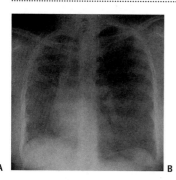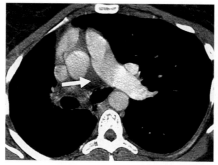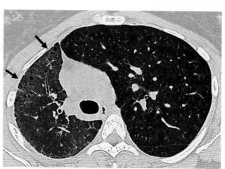

A   B   C

(A) Conventional chest radiograph shows asymmetric lung fields, with a smaller right hemithorax and ipsilateral deviation of the cardiac silhouette. **(B,C)** Contrast-enhanced computed tomography (CT) of the chest reveals absence of the right pulmonary artery and an asymmetric appearance of the lung parenchyma (*white arrow*, B). There are small, cystic-appearing changes in the periphery of the right lung, interlobular septal thickening, and a normal appearance of the left lung (*black arrows*, C).

■ Differential Diagnosis

- *Proximal interruption of the right pulmonary artery (PA):* Congenital absence of a PA with distal pulmonary vasculature in the affected side is consistent with the diagnosis of proximal interruption of the PA.
- *Pulmonary hypoplasia:* Imaging findings in pulmonary hypoplasia are similar, with diminished volume of the affected lung, but a PA, even a small one, should be apparent.
- *Hypogenetic lung syndrome:* In this condition, there is also reduced volume of the affected lung, typically the right, associated with an anomalous venous drainage of the right lung to the systemic circulation, but the PAs should be normal.

■ Essential Facts

- Proximal interruption of a PA is an uncommon anomaly that can occur on either side.
- This condition has also been referred to as unilateral absence of a PA, but it has been suggested that the term *interruption* is more appropriate because the distal pulmonary vasculature is not affected.
- The median age at diagnosis is 14 years.
- The clinical presentation includes dyspnea (40%), recurrent pulmonary infection (37%), and hemoptysis (20%).
- With interruption of the proximal PA, the pulmonary vasculature continues to develop and eventually receives oxygenated blood from systemic collaterals (e.g., bronchial arteries, intercostal arteries).

- In most cases, the interrupted PA is on the side opposite the aortic arch: absent right PA with a left-sided aortic arch and vice versa.
- Interruption of the PA is commonly associated with patent ductus arteriosus.
- Interruption of the left PA is commonly associated with tetralogy of Fallot, truncus arteriosus, and other congenital heart diseases.
- There is an abnormal prominence of the collateral systemic circulation, with large bronchial and intercostal arteries.
- Conventional chest radiography shows volume loss of the affected hemithorax with elevation of the ipsilateral hemidiaphragm and deviation of the heart and mediastinum to the affected side.
- There is an asymmetric appearance of the pulmonary hila, with one diminutive and the other more prominent. The contralateral lung is hyperinflated.

✓ Pearls & ✗ Pitfalls

- ✓ High-resolution CT of the lung parenchyma commonly demonstrates reticular opacities, septal thickening, cystic changes, and pleural thickening of the affected lung.
- ✗ In Swyer-James syndrome or McLeod syndrome (sequela of acute viral respiratory bronchiolitis in infancy or childhood), a single small or normal-size hyperlucent lung is appreciated but is characteristically associated with air trapping on expiratory images and bronchiectasis.

Case 6

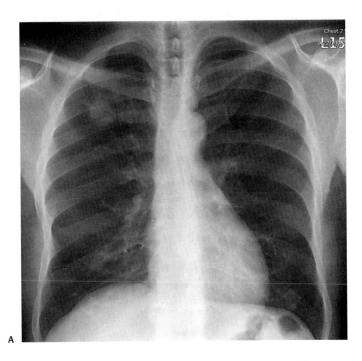

A

Clinical Presentation

A 57-year-old man with cough.

Further Work-up

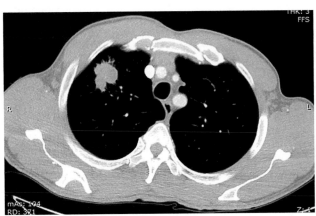

B

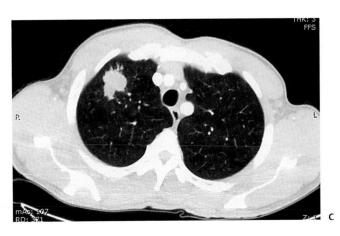

C

■ Imaging Findings

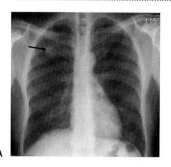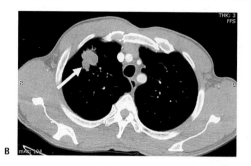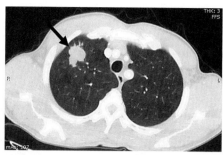

A   B   C

(A) Conventional radiograph of the chest reveals a lobulated, irregular 2.5-cm nodule in the right upper lobe (*arrow*). **(B,C)** Contrast-enhanced computed tomography (CT) images with mediastinal (B) and lung (C) windows confirm the presence of a spiculated, noncalcified, soft-tissue-density nodule in the anterior segment of the right upper lobe (*arrows*).

■ Differential Diagnosis

- **Lung cancer presenting as a solitary pulmonary nodule (SPN):** A spiculated, noncalcified pulmonary nodule in an adult patient should be considered lung cancer until proven otherwise.
- *Tuberculoma:* An active tuberculoma can present as a round, indeterminate pulmonary nodule, similar in appearance to lung cancer.
- *Round pneumonia:* Several infectious processes, bacterial or nonbacterial in etiology, may present as a round or spherical parenchymal consolidation in the form of an indeterminate SPN.

■ Essential Facts

- An SPN is defined as a focal, spherical (round or oval on imaging examinations) lesion in the lung parenchyma, surrounded by aerated lung, that measures less than 3 cm in diameter.
- A nodule that is not calcified in a benign pattern and that has not shown to be stable for longer than 2 years is referred to as an indeterminate nodule.
- An SPN may be detected on chest radiography or CT either in the evaluation of a symptomatic patient or as an incidental finding.
- A large number of benign and malignant conditions can present as an SPN.
- The majority of SPNs are benign, but depending on the patient's age, as many as 40% can be malignant.
- The most common cause of malignant SPN is adenocarcinoma (50%), followed by squamous cell carcinoma (25%).

- The most common causes of benign indeterminate SPN are nonspecific granulomas (25%), infectious granulomas (15%), and hamartomas (15%).
- One-fourth to one-third of lung cancers initially present as an SPN.
- The smaller the nodule, the greater the chance that it is benign; 80% of benign nodules are less than 2 cm in diameter.
- The likelihood of malignancy in nodules less than 5 mm in diameter is less than 1%.
- A lobulated contour reflects uneven growth and has been associated with malignancy.
- Nodules with an irregular or spiculated margin or a sunburst appearance (corona radiata sign) are more likely to be malignant.
- An air bronchogram within an SPN has also been associated with malignancy.
- Calcification is rare in lung cancers presenting as SPN (6%).
- Dynamic evaluation of nodule vascularity with CT has proved promising in the differentiation of benign from malignant indeterminate nodules. Enhancement of more than 25 Hounsfield units (HU; wash-in) favors malignancy, whereas absence of significant enhancement (< 15 HU) on CT favors a benign etiology.

✓ Pearls & ✗ Pitfalls

- ✓ The malignant SPN is a potentially curable form of lung cancer. More than 60 to 90% of patients with clinical stage IA (T1 N0 M0) cancers will be alive 5 years after diagnosis and treatment.
- ✗ More than half of nodules detected on conventional chest radiographs are false-positive findings and not confirmed on chest CT.

Case 7

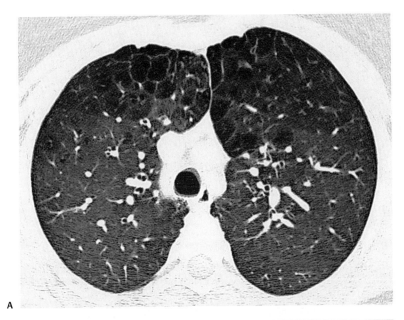

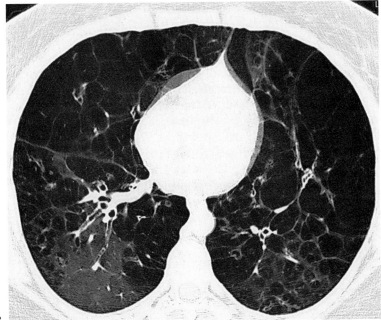

■ Clinical Presentation

A 26-year-old woman with progressive shortness of breath.

■ Imaging Findings

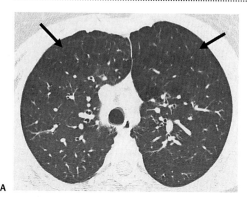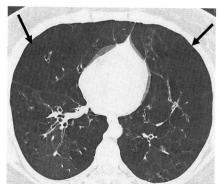

(A,B) High-resolution computed tomography of the chest: Axial images at the level of the upper lobes (A) and lower lung zones (B) demonstrate extensive emphysematous changes. Large bullous formations are seen bilaterally, more extensively involving the lower lung zones (*arrows*).

■ Differential Diagnosis

- *α₁-Antitrypsin (AAT) deficiency:* Panlobular emphysema, characterized by more extensive involvement of the lower lobes and lower segments in relatively young adults, is suggestive of AAT deficiency.
- *Centrilobular emphysema:* The typical distribution of centrilobular emphysema is upper lobe–predominant, and the characteristic morphology consists of smaller lucencies without a perceptible wall.
- *Cystic lung diseases:* Conditions like lymphangioleiomyomatosis and Langerhans cell histiocytosis may present with cystic changes of the lung, which manifest as thin-walled lucencies.

■ Essential Facts

- AAT deficiency is a hereditary condition in which absent or reduced serum levels of the AAT enzyme lead to the early development of pulmonary emphysema and effects on other organs and systems.
- AAT deficiency occurs in persons who inherit two protease inhibitor deficiency alleles of the AAT gene, located on chromosome 14.
- Panlobular (or panacinar) emphysema is the principal resulting clinical anomaly and the number one cause of morbidity and mortality in affected patients.
- In panlobular emphysema, the pulmonary lobules are uniformly destroyed from the level of the respiratory bronchioles to the level of the distal alveoli.
- The second most common and most significant clinical complication is liver disease (cholestasis and cirrhosis).

- Cirrhosis and carcinoma of the liver develop in up to 40% of patients with AAT deficiency who are older than 50 years of age.
- Smoking is the most significant additional risk factor for the rapid deterioration of pulmonary function in affected individuals.
- AAT deficiency should be suspected in subjects who have an early onset of emphysema (< 45 years of age), emphysema in the absence of recognized risk factors, emphysema with a predominantly lower lobe distribution, or emphysema with otherwise unexplained liver disease.
- The prevalence of AAT deficiency in the United States is about 1 in 3500 live births.
- Panlobular emphysema with basal predominance is the characteristic imaging finding. Associated centrilobular emphysema may be present in the upper lobes.
- Diffuse cystic bronchiectasis has been reported in 10 to 40% of patients with AAT deficiency.

✓ Pearls & ✗ Pitfalls

- ✓ The obstructive airway disease in AAT manifests on pulmonary function tests as a reduced ratio of the forced expiratory volume in 1 second to the forced vital capacity and is due mainly to the loss of elastic recoil as a consequence of parenchymal destruction.
- ✗ Panlobular emphysema is seen not only in patients with AAT deficiency but also in patients without AAT deficiency who smoke cigarettes, in whom panlobular emphysema may be associated with centrilobular emphysema.

Case 8

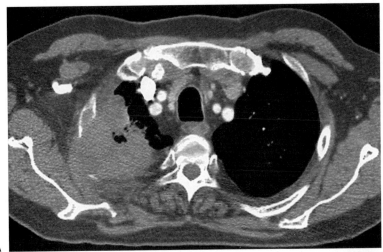

A

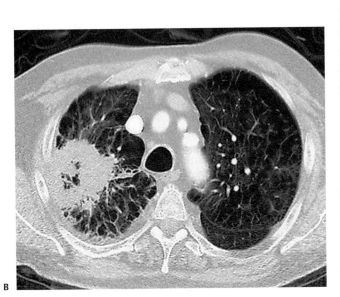

B

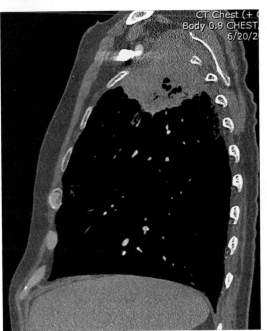

C

■ Clinical Presentation

A 68-year-old smoker with right shoulder pain, right arm weakness, cough, and abnormal symptoms in the right eye.

■ Imaging Findings

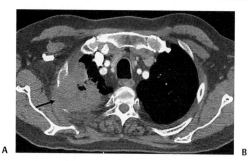
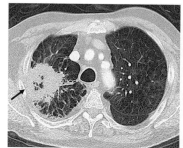
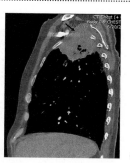

(A–C) Contrast-enhanced computed tomography (CT) of the chest demonstrates a large, spiculated soft-tissue mass with central areas of necrosis in the upper lobe of the right lung that extends to the pleura and chest wall (*arrows*). There is rib erosion and invasion of the superior sulcus. Extensive pulmonary emphysema is also noted.

■ Differential Diagnosis

- **Superior sulcus tumor (SST) and Pancoast syndrome:** A soft-tissue mass in the lung apex that presents with invasion of the chest wall and thoracic inlet is consistent with SST. The constellation of clinical findings reported in this patient corresponds to a Pancoast syndrome.
- *Bone tumor:* A primary bone tumor (e.g., osteosarcoma, plasmacytoma, lymphoma) or a secondary lesion (metastasis) may present as a neoplastic mass in the thoracic inlet with a soft-tissue component and associated bone erosion.
- *Pneumonia and osteomyelitis:* Rarely, an infectious process (e.g., tuberculosis, actinomycosis, aspergillosis) involving an upper lobe may extend to the chest wall and produce rib erosion and neurologic symptoms with a constellation of findings similar to those of a Pancoast syndrome.

■ Essential Facts

- SSTs (Pancoast tumors) are primary lung cancers, usually non–small-cell lung cancers, that occur in the apex of the lung and frequently invade the chest wall, first two or three upper ribs, vertebral bodies, and soft tissues of the thoracic inlet, including the subclavian vessels, brachial plexus, and stellate ganglion.
- According to cell type, the tumors are squamous cell carcinomas (40%), adenocarcinomas (20%), and anaplastic or poorly differentiated (25%). Small-cell carcinoma rarely presents in this way.
- Because they involve the chest wall, for staging purposes these tumors are considered to be T3 lesions. If there is mediastinal involvement (esophagus or trachea) or vertebral body involvement, they are considered to be T4 lesions.
- Approximately 3 to 5% of lung cancers present as an SST.

- Pancoast syndrome refers to a constellation of clinical findings, including shoulder and arm pain (typically along the distribution of the 8th cervical nerve trunk as well as the 1st and 2nd thoracic nerve trunks), Horner syndrome (ipsilateral myosis, ptosis, and anhidrosis), and weakness and atrophy of the muscles of the hand, that are secondary to local extension of a superior sulcus lung cancer.
- A unilateral apical cap larger than 5 mm in diameter, an apical mass, or bone erosion may be the initial imaging manifestation on conventional radiographs.
- Multidetector CT with multiplanar reconstruction better defines the epicenter of the mass in the lung parenchyma as well as chest wall involvement.

■ Other Imaging Findings

- Magnetic resonance imaging (MRI) is better than CT for the evaluation of chest wall involvement in lung cancers and is particularly good for the evaluation and staging of the thoracic inlet and SST. MRI better depicts involvement of the brachial plexus, neurovertebral foramina, and spinal canal.

✓ Pearls & ✗ Pitfalls

- ✓ In two classic papers in 1924 and 1932, radiologist Henry K. Pancoast (1875–1939) described the association of SST and Horner syndrome. Originally, he mistakenly believed that these tumors arose from embryologic nests of the 5th branchial cleft. The pulmonary origin of these tumors was later recognized by Pancoast and others.
- ✗ On plain films, SST can be difficult to detect. Subtle findings like a thick apical cap or soft-tissue mass may be confused with benign apical pleural thickening. Vertebral body or rib erosion can be difficult to detect on conventional radiographs.

Case 9

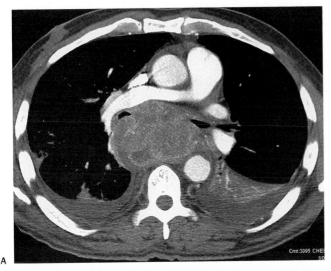

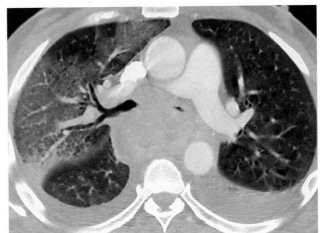

A   B

■ Clinical Presentation

A 58-year-old man with progressive dyspnea, cough, and dysphagia.

■ Imaging Findings

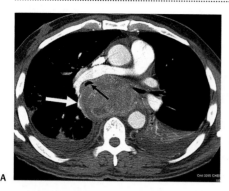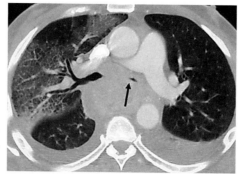

(A) Contrast-enhanced computed tomography (CT) shows a large mediastinal mass (*white arrow*) with heterogeneous enhancement, airway compression (*black arrows*), and bilateral pleural fluid collections. **(B)** Lung window image shows interlobular septal thickening and ground-glass opacity in the right lung.

■ Differential Diagnosis

- **Small-cell lung cancer (SCLC):** The most common imaging presentation is a large mediastinal mass, generally without imaging evidence of a lung parenchymal lesion.
- *Lymphoma:* A large mediastinal mass may also be the initial presentation of a lymphoma. The presence of airway obstruction helps in the differentiation between lymphoma and SCLC. Bronchial narrowing or an intraluminal mass is more common in lung cancer than in lymphoma.
- *Metastasis:* Various intrathoracic and extrathoracic malignancies with mediastinal dissemination may present as a large mediastinal mass.

■ Essential Facts

- Lung cancer is the most common type of cancer and the leading cause of cancer-related death in women and men worldwide.
- In the United States, more than 170,000 new cases are diagnosed each year.
- SCLC, also known as oat cell lung cancer, accounts for 20% of all primary lung cancers.
- Most SCLCs arise from the epithelium of the proximal airways (neuroendocrine cells), demonstrate rapid growth, and metastasize early.
- SCLCs are considered to be a type of neuroendocrine carcinoma.
- The incidence of SCLC is higher in males. SCLC occurs almost exclusively in cigarette smokers, and it usually presents at a younger age than non–small-cell lung cancer (NSCLC).
- Untreated, SCLC tends to be more aggressive than NSCLC. The prognosis is generally poor, with a 4% survival rate 5 years after diagnosis.
- The majority of patients have advanced disease at the time of diagnosis.

- Common imaging findings include a large, bulky mediastinal mass; a hilar mass; bronchial narrowing or obstruction; and post-obstructive pneumonitis.
- A minority of SCLCs (< 5%) present as limited disease (solitary pulmonary nodule).
- Common manifestations of SCLC include obstructive symptoms (cough, hemoptysis), dyspnea, dysphagia, hoarseness (recurrent laryngeal nerve involvement), and superior vena cava (SVC) syndrome.
- Positron emission tomography with 18F-fluorodeoxyglucose is superior to CT in the staging of SCLC and better identifies occult, advanced, or distant disease. This improved staging is critical in selecting appropriate treatment.
- Collateral circulation with prominent neck and chest wall veins may be seen in patients with SCLC presenting as SVC syndrome (12% of cases).

✓ Pearls & ✗ Pitfalls

- ✓ In the most common staging system for SCLC, the disease is classified as limited or extensive. Disease is considered to be limited when the tumor is confined to one hemithorax, the mediastinum, and one ipsilateral supraclavicular node. Disease is considered to be extensive if it is metastatic to the contralateral hemithorax or beyond the thorax, or if it cannot be encompassed by a single radiation port. Only 20% of patients have limited disease at the time of diagnosis.
- ✗ SCLC, like other neuroendocrine tumors, may produce metabolically active substances (e.g., adrenocorticotropic hormone, parathyroid hormone, antidiuretic hormone, and calcitonin) that manifest clinically before the lung cancer is diagnosed and create a confusing clinical scenario.

Case 10

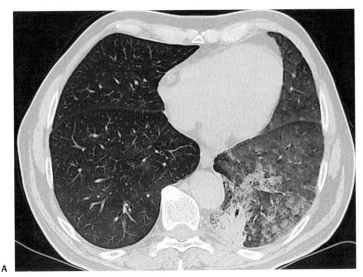

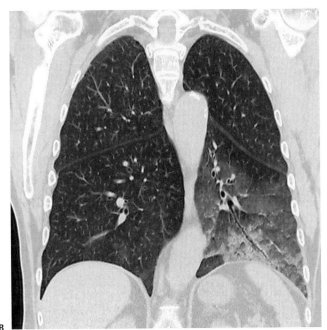

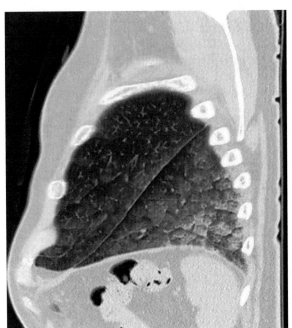

■ Clinical Presentation

A 49-year-old man with malaise and progressive cough for 1 month.

■ **Imaging Findings**

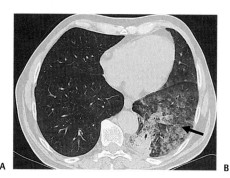
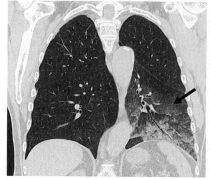
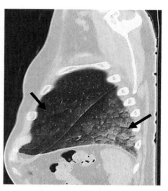

A B C

(A–C) Multidetector computed tomography (CT) axial (A), coronal (B), and sagittal (C) images. Extensive ground-glass opacity is appreciated in the left lower lobe and lingula, in some areas with a lobular distribution, and with a few patchy areas of denser air-space consolidation (*arrows*).

■ **Differential Diagnosis**

- ***Bronchioloalveolar carcinoma (BAC):*** In the differential diagnosis of pneumonia-like opacities in an adult, BAC should be considered.
- *Pneumonia:* The spectrum of infectious pneumonia can be quite variable, ranging from minimal parenchymal opacity to ill-defined ground-glass density to complete lobar or multifocal air-space consolidation. Atypical pneumonia (*Legionella pneumophila*, *Mycoplasma pneumoniae*, and *Chlamydophila pneumoniae*), as well as viral and pneumocystic pneumonia, may present as ground-glass opacities.
- *Interstitial pneumonia:* Some of the different types of interstitial pneumonia (desquamative interstitial pneumonia, nonspecific interstitial pneumonia) may present as extensive areas of ground-glass opacity. Other differential diagnoses include pulmonary edema, drug toxicity, and alveolar hemorrhage.

■ **Essential Facts**

- BAC is a particular subtype of adenocarcinoma of the lung characterized histologically by the spread of tumor cells on the peripheral air-space surface of the lung parenchyma. Tumor cells are arranged in a single layer without producing pulmonary architectural destruction (lepidic growth pattern).
- The incidence of this subtype of lung cancer has increased significantly in the last several decades. BACs account for fewer than 4% of all non–small-cell lung cancers (NSCLCs).
- BACs are divided into three types: mucinous, nonmucinous, and mixed or intermediate.

- The tumor cells may secrete intra-alveolar mucus or surfactant-like proteinaceous fluid, which can be quite significant in volume.
- The most common presentation of BAC is as a peripheral solitary pulmonary nodule (60%), followed by ill-defined areas of ground-glass opacity or consolidation, mimicking pneumonia.
- A BAC containing large amounts of mucin has low attenuation on CT.
- In the third and least common imaging pattern, BAC appears as multiple pulmonary nodules.
- The diffuse type of BAC is usually confused with pneumonia. Bronchial wall thickening proximal to the lesion and pleural thickening associated with the lesion favor pneumonia. Additionally, deformity of the air-filled bronchus within the area of parenchymal consolidation (stretching, squeezing, widening of the branching angle) or bulging of the interlobar fissure favors pneumonic-type BAC over infection.

✓ **Pearls & ✗ Pitfalls**

- ✓ The 1-year survival rate of patients with BAC is significantly better than that of patients with other histologic subtypes of NSCLC.
- ✗ Positron emission tomography with 18F-fluorodeoxyglucose has lower peak standardized uptake values and higher false-negative rates (40%) in BAC than in other NSCLC of the lungs. This lower sensitivity is more pronounced in the focal form of BAC than in multifocal BAC.

Case 11

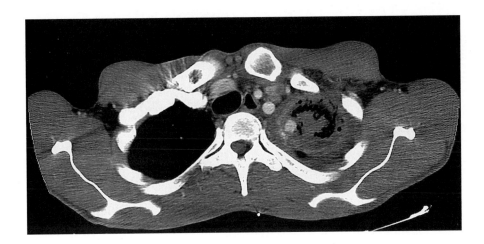

Clinical Presentation

A 43-year-old man with cough and hemoptysis.

■ Imaging Findings

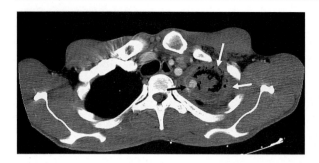

Contrast-enhanced computed tomography (CT): axial image at the level of the thoracic inlet shows a cavitary lesion in the left upper lobe with a crescent-shaped air density (*black arrow*), peripheral rim enhancement (*long white arrow*), and a round, denser area of vascular enhancement on its medial aspect (*short white arrow*).

■ Differential Diagnosis

- **Rasmussen aneurysm:** Infectious aneurysms in a pulmonary artery secondary to pulmonary tuberculosis (TB) are referred to as Rasmussen aneurysms. They characteristically develop as a result of weakening of a pulmonary artery wall adjacent to a TB cavity.
- *Infectious pulmonary aneurysm (mycotic aneurysm):* Mycotic aneurysms of a pulmonary artery result from septic pulmonary embolism, typically in patients with infective endocarditis, or from direct arterial wall involvement in patients with necrotizing pneumonia.
- *Traumatic pseudoaneurysm:* In patients who have sustained a penetrating lung injury, a traumatic pseudoaneurysm may develop in a peripheral pulmonary artery. Similarly, a pseudoaneurysm may develop secondary to endovascular injury from an intravascular catheter.

■ Essential Facts

- Hemoptysis in patients with TB may originate from either the bronchial arteries or the pulmonary arteries.
- Rasmussen aneurysms are pseudoaneurysms, considered to develop as a result of direct continuity with a focus of chronic fibrocaseous pulmonary parenchymal TB infection that directly invades or erodes a pulmonary artery.
- This mechanism is different from that seen in septic thromboembolism, in which the infective organism gains access to the arterial wall from a septic endovascular embolism that usually originates in an infected tricuspid valve in intravenous drug abusers.

- Localized dilatation of the medium-size pulmonary arteries contiguous with the fibrous capsule of the wall of a chronic TB cavity has been described in 4% of patients with chronic cavitary TB.
- Rasmussen aneurysms of the pulmonary arteries result from destruction of the media of segmental pulmonary arteries by infection-induced granulation tissue.

■ Other Imaging Findings

- Catheter angiography helps to delineate the origin of the bleeding when clinically significant hemoptysis develops as a complication of pulmonary TB. In addition, endovascular embolization may be used to control the hemorrhage.

✓ Pearls & ✗ Pitfalls

- ✓ Massive hemoptysis (> 300 mL/24 h) is a well-known complication of chronic cavitary TB and can be life-threatening in as many as 20% of cases.
- ✗ The role of contrast-enhanced CT may be limited in defining whether a pulmonary parenchymal aneurysm or pseudoaneurysm originates from the pulmonary arterial circulation or from the bronchial systemic vasculature.

Case 12

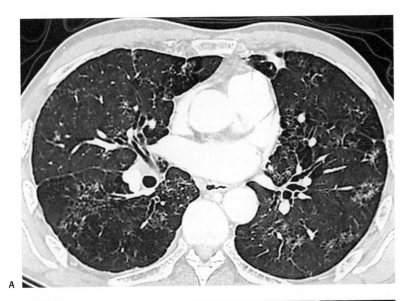

A

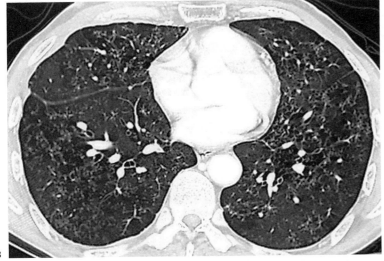

B

■ Clinical Presentation

A previously healthy 39-year-old man with a worsening productive cough for 3 months.

■ Imaging Findings

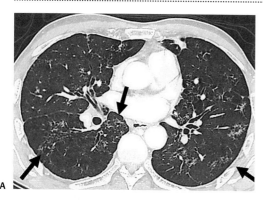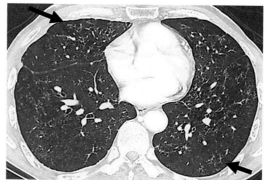

(A,B) Computed tomography (CT) of the chest demonstrates small nodular and branching irregular opacities throughout both lungs (*arrows*).

■ Differential Diagnosis

- ***Tuberculosis (TB) with bronchogenic spread:*** An imaging pattern of disease better seen on high-resolution CT, the tree-in-bud (TIB) pattern is characterized by small, centrilobular nodules interconnected through linear branching structures. It is commonly seen in infectious or inflammatory conditions of the lung, in particular TB infection with bronchogenic spread.
- *Other infections:* Atypical mycobacterial infection (*Mycobacterium avium–intracellulare* complex), fungal infection (aspergillosis), and occasionally viral infection (cytomegalovirus infection) may present with centrilobular nodules and branching opacities that have a TIB pattern.
- *Cystic fibrosis:* The mucous plugging seen in cystic fibrosis may also present with a TIB pattern. Additional findings in these patients include cylindric bronchiectasis and bronchial wall thickening, which tend to affect the upper lobes more significantly.

■ Essential Facts

- The TIB pattern seen on thin-section CT represents bronchiolar impaction and dilation with intraluminal pus, mucus, fluid, or inflammatory exudate, which fills the small-caliber peripheral airways and makes them visible on imaging examinations.
- On histologic examination, dilatation and wall thickening, in addition to bronchiolar and peribronchiolar inflammation, are identified.

- The TIB pattern is a nonspecific sign of bronchiolar disease.
- This imaging sign is commonly, but not exclusively, seen in cases of TB with bronchogenic spread.
- In general, the majority of diseases that present with the TIB pattern are infectious or inflammatory conditions, or they are disorders associated with postinfectious bronchiectasis.
- Other infectious processes, such as bacterial infection, atypical mycobacterial infection, aspergillosis, and viral and parasitic infection, may present with similar imaging findings.
- Other diseases of the small airways (e.g., diffuse panbronchiolitis and obliterative panbronchiolitis), as well as congenital disorders such as cystic fibrosis and primary ciliary dyskinesia, may also present with this imaging finding.
- Additional signs of bronchiolar obstruction, such as air trapping, may be seen in patients with the TIB pattern.

✓ Pearls & ✗ Pitfalls

- ✓ When the TIB pattern is found in a patient with pulmonary TB, it represents the bronchial spread of caseous material and favors an active infection.
- ✗ TIB opacities may not be visible on conventional chest radiographs.

Case 13

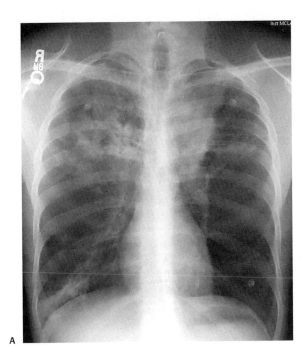

A

■ Clinical Presentation

A 29-year-old man with a long history of asthma and a productive cough.

Further Work-up

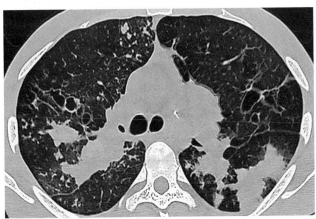

B

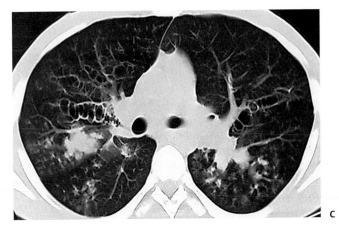

C

■ Imaging Findings

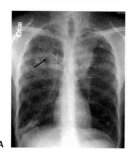 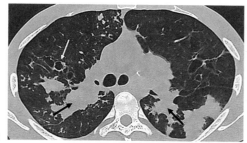 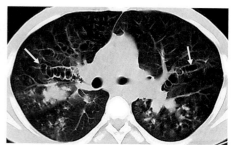

(A) Radiograph of the chest shows ill-defined, multifocal parenchymal opacities bilaterally that are more confluent in the upper lobes. Irregular, elongated tubular densities are better appreciated on the right side (*arrow*). **(B,C)** Computed tomography (CT) of the chest with lung window images reveals cylindric bronchiectasis (*white arrows*) and the irregular tubular structure radiating from the hilar region to the periphery of the right lung (*black arrows*). Areas of tree-in-bud (TIB) opacity in the periphery of both lungs are also identified

■ Differential Diagnosis

- ***Allergic bronchopulmonary aspergillosis (ABPA):*** Finger-like shadows in a bronchial distribution are the characteristic finding of ABPA. The shadows represent mucus plugs, more significantly involving the upper lobes, as well as bronchiectasis, and are occasionally associated with atelectasis.
- *Cystic fibrosis:* Bronchiectasis with mucoid impaction is relatively common in patients with cystic fibrosis. Usually, other findings, such as bronchiolar impaction (TIB opacities), emphysema, abscess, and bullous formations, are also present.
- *Bronchial atresia:* Mucoid impaction associated with bronchial atresia is common but characteristically involves a single lobe or segment.

■ Essential Facts

- ABPA results from a hypersensitivity reaction to *Aspergillus* organisms, in particular *A. fumigatus.*
- The fungus does not invade tissue (bronchial or pulmonary).
- Marked local and systemic eosinophilia is characteristic of this condition.
- ABPA is a complication of persistent asthma (1–2%) and cystic fibrosis (5–15%), in part related to the excessive production of viscous mucus and abnormal mucociliary clearance.

- Inhaled *Aspergillus* spores colonize and multiply in pre-existing mucus, inducing an allergic reaction with increased inflammation and further production of mucus.
- Histopathology reveals central bronchiectasis, eosinophilic pneumonitis, bronchocentric granulomatosis, bronchiolitis, and hyphae-laden microabscesses.
- Clinical manifestations include chronic cough, bronchorrhea, brown plugs containing *Aspergillus* hyphae in the sputum, and wheezing.
- Imaging findings include central bronchiectasis (> 80%), which is predominant in the upper lobes, toothpaste or gloved-finger mucoid impaction, and pulmonary consolidation, which may represent eosinophilic alveolar infiltrates (eosinophilic pneumonia).
- Atelectasis due to retained secretions, which tend to shift over time from one part of the lung to another and may be segmental or lobar or affect an entire lung, is an additional finding commonly seen in ABPA.

✓ Pearls & ✗ Pitfalls

- ✓ In some patients with ABPA (25%), the inspissated mucous plugs in the dilated bronchi may on CT have a density higher than that expected for soft tissues. Similarly, high-density material is known to occur in the sinuses of patients with chronic allergic fungal sinusitis.
- ✗ The sensitivity of plain films for the detection of bronchiectasis, which is one of the most significant features of ABPA, is limited (50%). Thin-slice CT should always be used to detect this abnormal finding.

Case 14

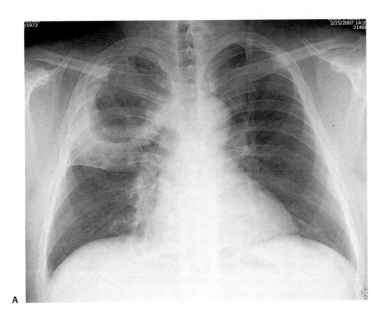

A

■ Clinical Presentation

A 34-year-old man with fever, productive cough, and malaise 1 week after being hospitalized for diabetic ketoacidosis.

Further Work-up

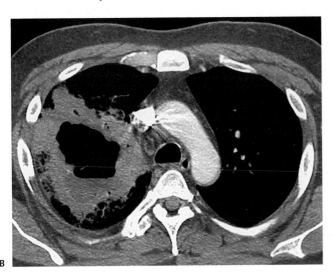

B

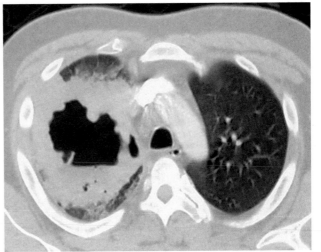

C

■ Imaging Findings

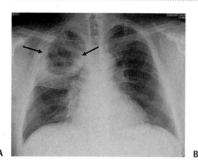
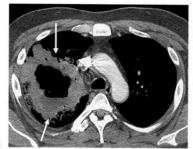
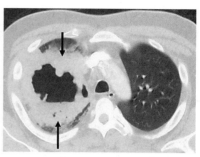

(A) Conventional radiograph of the chest shows a parenchymal opacity in the right upper lobe with a central area of cavitation (*arrows*). **(B,C)** Contrast-enhanced computed tomography of the chest confirms the presence of air-space consolidation in the posterior segment of the right upper lobe with central, thick-walled cavitation (*arrows*).

■ Differential Diagnosis

- **Klebsiella *pneumonia:*** This Gram-negative bacillus, as well as other Gram-negative organisms (*Escherichia coli* and *Pseudomonas aeruginosa*), are important causes of nosocomial pneumonia and are more likely than other organisms to cause necrotizing disease and cavity formation.
- *Tuberculosis:* Reactivation tuberculosis also tends to involve the posterior segment of the upper lobes and to present with necrosis and cavitation. Lobar consolidation of the surrounding parenchyma is less common.
- *Necrotizing lung cancer:* In adults, lung cancer should always be considered in the differential diagnosis of a cavitary lesion of the upper lobes, especially if it is thick-walled. Similarly, as discussed previously, surrounding air-space lobar consolidation is more common in necrotizing pneumonia than in malignancy.

■ Essential Facts

- Gram-negative bacilli, including *Klebsiella pneumoniae, P. aeruginosa, Enterobacter,* and *E. coli,* are important causes of nosocomial and community-acquired pneumonia.
- With some variation among medical centers, the most common pathogens isolated in patients with nosocomial pneumonia are Gram-negative organisms (60%) and *Staphylococcus aureus* (15%).
- Important risk factors include intubation, mechanical ventilation, enteral nutrition, reduced level of consciousness, and increased gastric pH (achlorhydria or the administration of antacids, histamine blockers, or other antacid medication), among others.
- Between 50 and 70% of cases of ventilator-associated nosocomial pneumonia in intensive care units are caused by Gram-negative bacilli.

- *Klebsiella pneumoniae* is the most common infective agent seen in the elderly, alcoholics, and debilitated men.
- The source of pulmonary infection is commonly aspirated infected oral secretions.
- The infectious process typically involves the posterior segment of the right upper lobe or the posterior lower lobes.
- Parapneumonic pleural effusion and empyema are common complications in these patients (> 60%).
- Lobar consolidation is more typical of *Klebsiella* pneumonia, whereas bronchopneumonia, manifesting as multifocal opacities (80%), is more common with *E. coli* and *P. aeruginosa* infection.
- *Klebsiella* pneumonia tends to present with lobar expansion and bulging of the interlobar fissures (30%) more than with pneumococcal consolidation (10%). This finding is known as the bulging fissure sign.

✓ Pearls & ✗ Pitfalls

- ✓ Pneumatoceles differ from lung abscesses associated with Gram-negative or anaerobic bacteria.
- ✓ Pneumatoceles are thin-walled, gas-filled spaces seen in areas of air-space disease and consolidation in patients with pneumonia. They develop from the acute infection and resolve in weeks or months.
- ✓ Pneumatoceles represent a form of lung abscess and are more commonly seen in children with *S. aureus* infection. A check-valve mechanism producing airway obstruction and air trapping is part of the pathophysiology and explains the transient nature of this finding.
- ✗ Partially resolved *Klebsiella* pneumonia, in which the bulk of the consolidation resolves, leaving an upper lobe cavity and scarring, may have imaging findings similar to those seen in reactivation tuberculosis.

Case 15

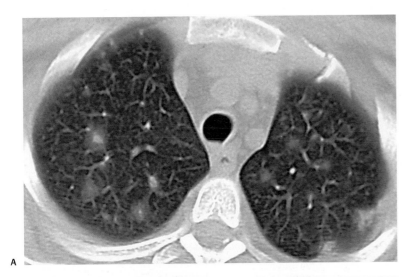

A

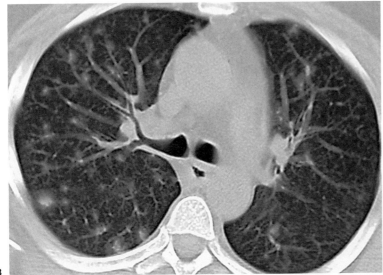

B

◼ Clinical Presentation

A 38-year-old man with skin rash, shortness of breath, cough, and fever.

■ Imaging Findings

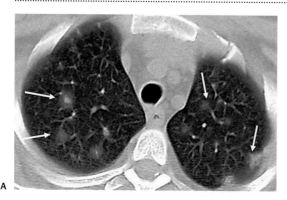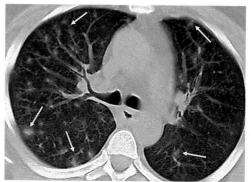

A   B

(A,B) Computed tomography of the chest without contrast reveals ill-defined ground-glass nodules scattered throughout both lungs (*arrows*). No lobar consolidation, no pleural effusion, and no enlarged lymph nodes are noted.

■ Differential Diagnosis

- **Varicella pneumonia:** The association of the typical skin rash with multiple pulmonary nodules scattered throughout the lung parenchyma should raise the question of varicella-zoster virus pneumonia.
- *Other viral pneumonias (cytomegalovirus [CMV] pneumonia, influenza virus pneumonia, measles):* Several viral pneumonias in adult patients may present with a combination of irregular patchy opacities and nodular ground-glass densities in the lung parenchyma.
- *Hemorrhagic pulmonary metastasis:* Hemorrhagic pulmonary metastasis from choriocarcinoma or angiosarcoma may present as multiple ground-glass pulmonary nodules.

■ Essential Facts

- Viral pneumonias in adult patients may present in two different clinical settings: in an otherwise healthy host (so-called atypical pneumonia) or in an immunocompromised host.
- The proportion of viral infections in cases of community-acquired pneumonia varies from 10 to 50%, depending on the age of the population, geography, and diagnostic criteria.
- Common viral infectious agents in immunocompetent hosts includes influenza viruses A and B, adenoviruses, Epstein-Barr virus, and hantaviruses.
- The most common viral infectious agents in immunocompromised patients include CMV, herpes simplex viruses, varicella-zoster virus, measles virus, and adenoviruses.

- Imaging manifestations in viral pneumonias usually reflect the combination of interstitial and air-space disease, with multifocal, poorly defined areas of patchy consolidation, ground-glass opacities, centrilobular nodules, reticular opacities resulting from interlobular septal thickening, and lobular consolidation.
- Lobar consolidation is less common in viral pneumonia than in bacterial infection.
- Interstitial opacities can be seen in both bacterial and viral pneumonias.
- The differentiation between bacterial and viral pneumonias on clinical grounds or laboratory findings is limited; the proportions of patients with an elevated white cell count or elevated erythrosedimentation rate are similar in bacterial and viral pneumonias.
- In some viral pneumonias, particularly in children, significant bronchial wall thickening with overinflation and atelectasis is the dominant imaging finding.

✓ Pearls & ✗ Pitfalls

- ✓ Pneumonia is a common and serious complication of varicella-zoster infection (chickenpox) in adults, with significant morbidity and mortality.
- ✗ Pleural effusion is not exclusively a complication of bacterial pneumonias. A significant amount of parapneumonic pleural fluid can be associated with different types of viral pneumonia.

Case 16

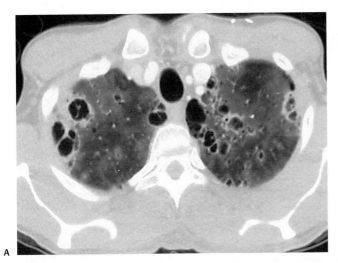

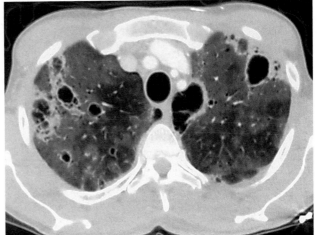

A

B

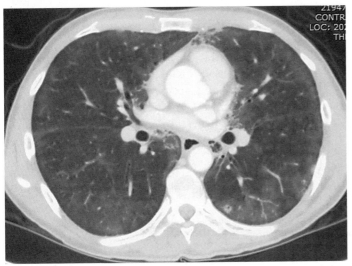

C

■ Clinical Presentation

A 44-year-old man with acquired immunodeficiency syndrome, now presenting with progressive cough and shortness of breath.

■ Imaging Findings

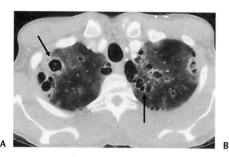 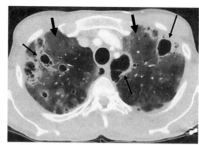 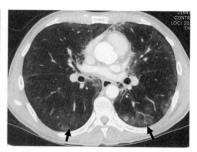

(A–C) Contrast-enhanced computed tomography (CT) axial images at three different levels reveal ill-defined multifocal areas of ground-glass opacity in both lungs (*thick arrows*) with irregular cysts in the upper lobes (*thin arrows*).

■ Differential Diagnosis

- **Pneumocystis** *pneumonia:* Multifocal ground-glass opacities that are more confluent in the upper lobes associated with cystic changes in a patient with acquired immunodeficiency syndrome (AIDS) is one of the imaging manifestations of *Pneumocystis* pneumonia.
- *Cytomegalovirus pneumonia:* Ground-glass opacities with a multifocal distribution may also be seen in immunocompromised patients with cytomegalovirus infection. Associated findings include pulmonary nodules.
- *Pulmonary edema:* Diffuse ground-glass opacity and interlobular septal thickening are very common imaging findings in pulmonary edema.

■ Essential Facts

- *Pneumocystis* pneumonia is an infection caused by *Pneumocystis jiroveci*, an opportunistic fungal pathogen.
- *Pneumocystis* is the most prevalent opportunistic infectious agent in patients who test positive for human immunodeficiency virus (HIV). It is responsible for 25% of cases of pneumonia in HIV patients and one of the most common causes of death among patients with AIDS.
- Affected patients typically have profound T-cell immunosuppression, with a CD4-cell count of less than 200/mm³.
- Affected patients often present with fever, nonproductive cough, dyspnea, hypoxemia, and elevated lactic dehydrogenase levels.
- Bilateral diffuse or multifocal ground-glass opacities are a characteristic finding.

- When the ground-glass opacities are associated with interlobular septal thickening, crazy-paving is the dominant imaging pattern.
- Severe cases may present with dense air-space consolidation.
- CT reveals ground-glass opacities in the parahilar regions and in the upper lobe of both lungs.
- Pleural effusion and lymphadenopathy are uncommon findings in *Pneumocystis* pneumonia.
- *P. jiroveci* infection less commonly presents in patients with forms of immunosuppression other than AIDS, such as transplant recipients (10%), patients with solid tumors, and patients with collagen vascular disease receiving steroid therapy (2%).
- Pulmonary cysts, one of the complications of *Pneumocystis* infection (10–30%), may result in spontaneous pneumothorax.
- *P. jiroveci* pneumonia demonstrates increased activity on nuclear medicine gallium scan.

✓ Pearls & ✗ Pitfalls

- ✓ *Pneumocystis* infection in humans is produced by *P. jiroveci*, which is different from *Pneumocystis carinii*. *P. carinii* causes infections in mammals others than human beings.
- ✗ *Pneumocystis* is a well-known cause of proven pneumonia in patients with normal findings on chest radiographs (10–30%), but it is extremely rare for patients with *Pneumocystis* pneumonia to have normal findings on high-resolution CT scans of the lungs.

Case 17

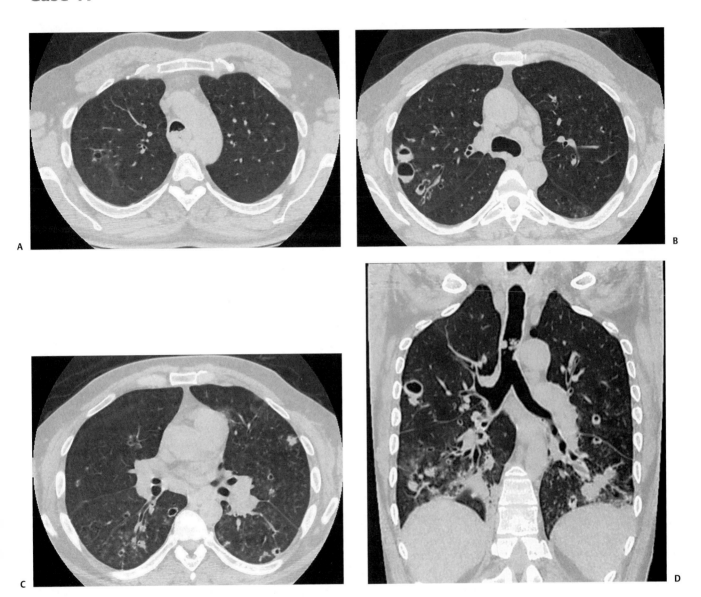

A

B

C

D

■ Clinical Presentation

A young man with progressive shortness of breath, hoarseness, chronic cough, and a past medical history of endobronchial resection of a tracheal mass.

■ Imaging Findings

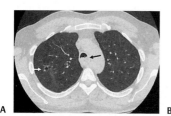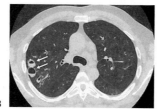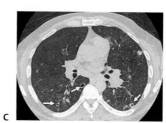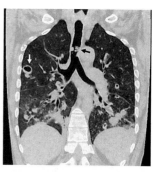

(A–D) Computed tomography of the chest: Axial images at three different levels (A–C) and coronal reconstruction (D). An irregular cauliflowerlike mass is seen partially obstructing the tracheal lumen (*black arrows*). Numerous nodules, cysts, and tree-in-bud and irregular patchy opacities are appreciated in the lower lobes of both lungs (*white arrows*). Left hilar lymphadenopathy is also noted.

■ Differential Diagnosis

- ***Tracheobronchial papillomatosis:*** The combination of an endoluminal tracheal mass, cavitating and noncavitating pulmonary nodules, and tree-in-bud opacities is characteristic of tracheobronchial papillomatosis.
- *Pneumatoceles in staphylococcal or Gram-negative pneumonia:* Pneumatoceles are common in patients with staphylococcal pulmonary infection (60%). They form in areas of pneumonic consolidation, presenting as pulmonary cysts.
- *Autoimmune disease:* Autoimmune diseases, such as rheumatoid arthritis with necrobiotic nodules, Wegener granulomatosis, and rarely polyarteritis nodosa, may present with cavitary nodules in the lung parenchyma.

■ Essential Facts

- Tracheobronchial papillomatosis is caused by human papillomavirus infection (types 6 and 11), usually acquired at birth (vertical transmission) from an infected mother with genital papillomas.
- The most common location for the airway infection is the larynx, from which the infection may spread distally to the trachea, bronchi, and rarely the lung parenchyma.
- The majority of cases present in childhood, before the age of 5 years.
- Laryngeal involvement occurs in almost all patients, whereas tracheal involvement occurs in a minority of cases (3–25%).
- Pulmonary parenchymal disease is even less common, reported in fewer than 3% of affected patients, more commonly in males.

- The virus induces a papillary proliferation of epithelial (squamous) cells, which projects into the lumen of the affected airways. Tracheobronchial papillomatosis may present either as a focal mass or as a diffuse cobblestone appearance of the mucosa.
- Aerial dissemination of the virus and a lepidic pattern of squamous cell spread may occur.
- The imaging appearance consists of multiple pulmonary nodules, usually small (< 1 cm), that may cavitate as they progress and enlarge.
- The cavity walls are usually thin.
- Endobronchial papillomatosis may give a nodular appearance to the airways.
- Patients with laryngotracheal disease often require multiple endoluminal procedures to maintain a patent airway.
- Atelectasis and postobstructive pneumonitis may develop distal to endobronchial obstructive papillomas.

✓ Pearls & ✗ Pitfalls

- ✓ Malignant transformation into squamous or adenosquamous cell carcinoma has been reported in both juvenile and adult patients and may present as multicentric tumor.
- ✗ It is important always to check the trachea carefully in patients with multiple cystic or cavitary lesions in the lung parenchyma. Laryngotracheal or bronchial papillomas may be small and subtle.

Case 18

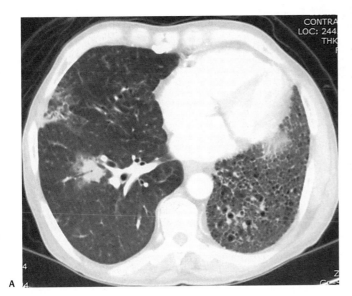 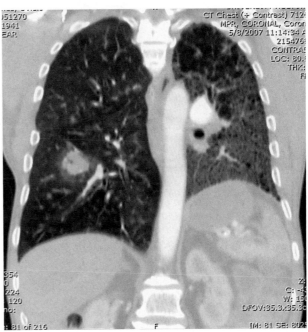

Clinical Presentation

A 66-year-old man who has received a right-sided lung transplant for pulmonary fibrosis presents with right-sided chest pain, fever, and cough.

■ Imaging Findings

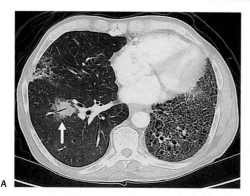
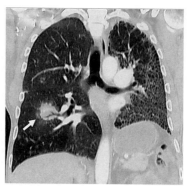

A

B

(A,B) Contrast-enhanced computed tomography (CT): Axial (A) and coronal (B) images demonstrate a focal area of air-space nodular consolidation in the right lower lobe, surrounded by a ground-glass halo of lesser density. An irregular wedge-shaped opacity in the periphery of the middle lobe is also seen (*arrows*). There is end-stage fibrosis of the left lung.

■ Differential Diagnosis

- ***Angioinvasive aspergillosis with the halo sign:*** In an immunosuppressed patient, a dense nodule surrounded by a ground-glass halo is highly suggestive of angioinvasive aspergillosis.
- *Hemorrhagic tumor:* Neoplastic conditions may also present with a dense nodule or mass surrounded by a ground-glass rim.
- *Vasculitis:* Pulmonary changes secondary to vasculitis may also manifest with a central dense nodular opacity and a peripheral halo. Clinical correlation is important to differentiate among the various conditions that may exhibit a halo sign.

■ Essential Facts

- The halo sign consists of a halo of ground-glass attenuation, which represents alveolar hemorrhage, surrounding a central denser nodule, which corresponds to a focus of infarction.
- This imaging sign was originally described in patients with invasive aspergillosis.
- In immunosuppressed patients, in particular neutropenic patients, the halo sign is suggestive of aspergillosis, mucormycosis (*Rhizopus*), candidiasis, coccidioidomycosis, or infection with other fungi.
- In particular, angioinvasive fungi (*Aspergillus* and *Mucor*) should be suspected in neutropenic patients with this finding.
- The prevalence of the halo sign varies with the evolution of the disease. It is more prevalent (> 90%) during the first days, early in the course of the disease, and less prevalent (< 20%) after 2 weeks.

- Approximately half of the nodules may evolve to cavitation.
- Risk factors for angioinvasive aspergillosis include immunosuppression with severe neutropenia after treatment for hematologic malignancies (high-dose chemotherapy, stem cell transplant, or bone marrow transplant), as well as immunosuppression after solid organ transplant and the use of corticosteroids to treat autoimmune diseases.
- Besides nodules, angioinvasive aspergillosis may also manifest as wedge-shaped areas of peripheral parenchymal consolidation.

■ Other Imaging Findings

- High-resolution multidetector row CT pulmonary angiography may help in differentiating among various conditions presenting with the halo sign by detecting vascular occlusion in angioinvasive aspergillosis.

✓ Pearls & ✗ Pitfalls

✓ Angioinvasive pulmonary aspergillosis has a high morbidity and mortality rate (> 30%) in immunocompromised patients.

✗ Besides opportunistic infection, the halo sign has been demonstrated in other conditions associated with pulmonary hemorrhage, including metastasis (angiosarcoma, choriocarcinoma), Kaposi sarcoma, vasculitis, organizing pneumonia, and lung injury.

Case 19

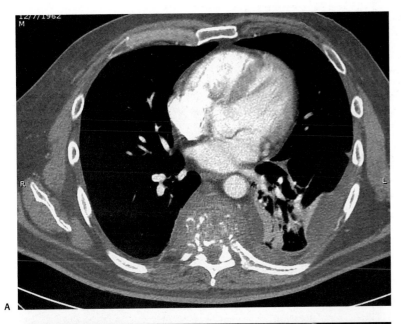

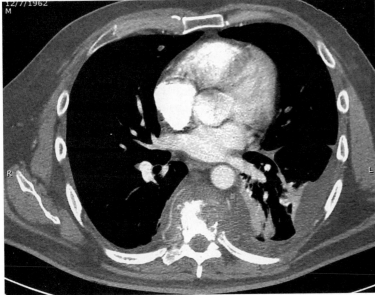

▪ Clinical Presentation

A 44-year-old male intravenous drug abuser with hepatitis C and acquired immunodeficiency syndrome, now presenting with progressive back and chest pain.

Imaging Findings

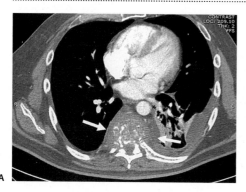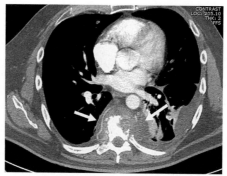

(A,B) Contrast-enhanced computed tomography (CT) shows an osteolytic lesion and fluid density involving the lower thoracic spine (*arrows*), with a paraspinal low-density mass displacing the aorta and other vessels anteriorly, as well as a left-sided pleural effusion.

Differential Diagnosis

- **Bacterial spondylodiskitis (vertebral osteomyelitis):** Vertebral body destruction and paraspinal fluid (abscess) are characteristic findings of bacterial infection of the vertebral bodies and disk.
- *Osteolytic tumor:* Primary (e.g., plasmacytoma, lymphoma) or secondary (e.g., metastasis from lung cancer, breast cancer) tumors may also present as vertebral body erosion, pathologic fracture, and paraspinal bleeding.
- *Vertebral body fracture:* Trauma with vertebral body fracture may present with paraspinal and posterior mediastinal hematoma.

Essential Facts

- Bacterial spondylodiskitis is the infection of an intervertebral disk space and the adjacent vertebral bodies.
- The infectious process is believed to begin at the vertebral body end plate as the consequence of hematogenous dissemination from a distant source (urinary tract infection, skin, prostatitis, endocarditis).
- Important risk factors include intravenous drug abuse, diabetes, malnutrition, renal failure, steroid therapy, human immunodeficiency virus infection, and other causes of immunosuppression.
- *Staphylococcus aureus* accounts for more than 50% of cases of pyogenic spondylodiskitis.
- Other infectious microorganisms include *Streptococcus viridans, Escherichia coli, Staphylococcus epidermidis,* and other Gram-negative bacteria, such as *Proteus* and *Pseudomonas.*
- In some parts of the world, *Mycobacterium tuberculosis* is still a common cause of spinal infection (Pott disease), second only to *Staphylococcus aureus.*
- Clinical manifestations include back pain (90%), fever, night sweats, anemia, and, in advanced stages, neurologic manifestations of spinal cord compression.

- The thoracic or thoracolumbar spine is affected in nearly 45% of cases.
- Compression fractures and epidural abscess may result in significant neurologic complications of spinal cord compression.
- One in every three or four cases is complicated by an epidural abscess.
- Conventional radiography may reveal collapse of a vertebral body or an intervertebral disk space.
- CT may show more obvious vertebral body destruction, disk space obliteration, and paraspinal abscess.
- Typical findings of spondylodiskitis on magnetic resonance imaging (MRI) are low signal intensity of the disks and adjacent vertebral bodies on T1-weighted images and hyperintensity on T2-weighted and fat-suppressed sequences.

Other Imaging Findings

- Contrast-enhanced MRI shows inhomogeneous enhancement of the disks and adjacent vertebral bodies, and of the epidural and paravertebral soft tissue. Enhancing areas represent granulation tissue, whereas nonenhancing areas represent necrosis and abscess formation. Pathologic intraspinal and paravertebral soft-tissue and epidural abscess, when present, can also be better appreciated with contrast-enhanced MRI.

✓ Pearls & ✗ Pitfalls

- ✓ MRI is the imaging modality of choice for the diagnosis of infective spondylodiskitis, particularly in the early stages of the disease, when other imaging modalities yield negative results.
- ✗ In the early stage of infective spondylodiskitis, the findings on conventional radiography and CT may be normal.

Case 20

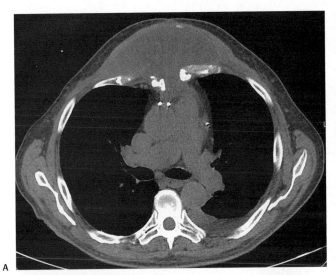

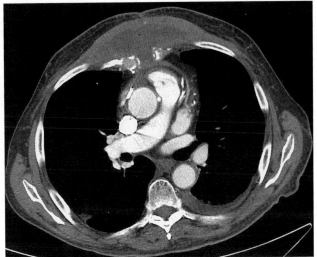

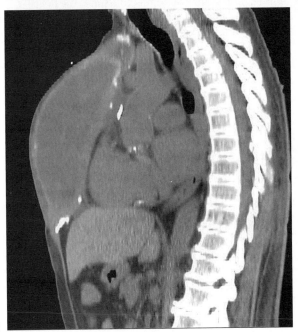

■ Clinical Presentation

A patient who has undergone revascularization surgery, now presenting with chest pain, swelling of the anterior chest wall, and fever.

■ Imaging Findings

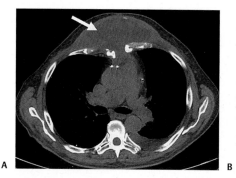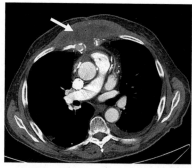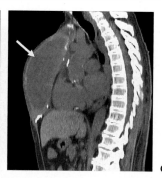

A   B   C

(A–C) Axial noncontrast-enhanced (A) and contrast-enhanced (B) images and noncontrast-enhanced sagittal reconstruction (C) show full-length, midline sternotomy dehiscence. A large, low-density fluid collection in the presternal region of the anterior chest wall is in continuity with the anterior mediastinum (*arrows*).

■ Differential Diagnosis

- *Poststernotomy dehiscence, infection, and abscess:* In a patient with fever and pain who has previously undergone surgical sternotomy, a presternal fluid collection and sternal wound dehiscence, with or without mediastinal fluid, are consistent with infection.
- *Poststernotomy hematoma or seroma:* Sternal wound dehiscence may also present with uninfected fluid collections, such as hematomas or seromas. Hematomas usually present with high density.
- *Lymphangioma:* Fluid collections in the anterior chest wall may be seen in patients with lymphangiomas. They are usually not associated with fever, are congenital in nature, and are not related to sternal surgery.

■ Essential Facts

- Dehiscence and infection of median sternotomy wounds occur in up to 5% of cases.
- This complication has been associated with increased mortality in the past (14–47%), in particular in patients with underlying mediastinitis. Currently, the mortality rate has decreased (< 10%) but remains high.
- Preoperative risk factors include diabetes mellitus, obesity, smoking, chronic obstructive pulmonary disease, and larger female breast size.
- Perioperative risk factors are prolonged bypass time and suboptimal sternal closure.
- Postoperative risk factors include transfusions, surgical re-exploration, prolonged postoperative ventilation, positive wound culture, and tracheotomy.
- Whether harvesting of the internal mammary arteries is associated with sternal devascularization and subsequently an increased rate of wound complications (dehiscence and infection) is still a matter of debate.
- Imaging findings on conventional radiographs may

demonstrate ruptured wires, sternal dehiscence, and wire malposition.
- Computed tomography better demonstrates the dehiscence, changes in bone density or morphology, and fluid collections in the anterior chest wall, wound, or anterior mediastinum.
- Fluid collections may occasionally contain gas bubbles.
- *Staphylococcus aureus* is the most common pathogen in sternal wound infections (30%), followed by *Staphylococcus epidermidis* (20%).
- Superficial infection is treated with simple incision, drainage, and antibiotic therapy. Deep sternal wound infection additionally requires sternal and soft-tissue debridement and surgical closure.

■ Other Imaging Findings

- The role of radionuclide imaging is controversial. A prospective study suggested that radionuclide scanning with gallium 67 has a high sensitivity (83%) and specificity (96%) for the diagnosis of sternal osteomyelitis.

✓ Pearls & ✗ Pitfalls

- ✓ With dehiscence, sternal wires are seen displaced to either side of the chest as they are pulled through the sternum (> 2 cm), rather than fracture. Sternal wire breaks per se are not indicative of dehiscence or infection.
- ✗ A midsternal lucent stripe seen on conventional radiographs is not a reliable indicator of dehiscence or infection.

Case 21

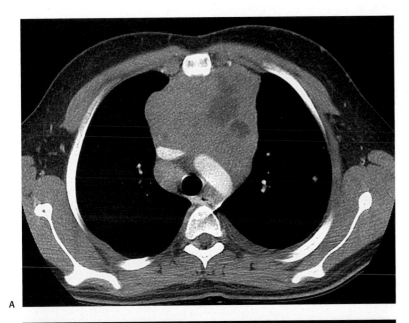

A

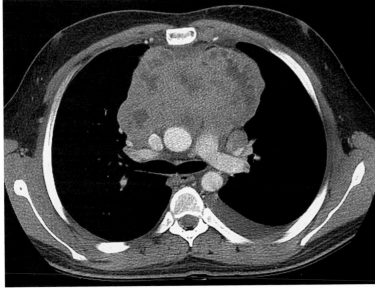

B

■ Clinical Presentation

A 29-year-old man with malaise, fever, and fatigue.

■ Imaging Findings

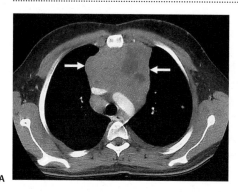
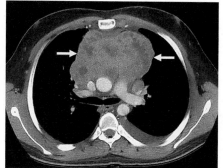

A   **B**

(A,B) Contrast-enhanced computed tomography (CT): Axial images at two different levels. There is a large heterogeneous mass in the anterior mediastinum, with enlarged mediastinal and hilar lymph nodes and a left-sided pleural effusion (*arrows*).

■ Differential Diagnosis

- **Lymphoma (diffuse large B-cell):** A large mass in the anterior mediastinum associated with enlarged hilar lymph nodes or lymphadenopathy in other mediastinal compartments is a common presentation of mediastinal lymphoma.
- *Germ cell tumor:* Germ cell tumors commonly present as soft-tissue-density mass in the anterior mediastinum.
- *Thymoma:* Thymomas and masses derived from the thyroid gland also present as anterior mediastinal mass.

■ Essential Facts

- Lymphoma accounts for ~4% of new cancers diagnosed in the United States each year and is the fifth leading cause of cancer-related deaths.
- Both Hodgkin lymphoma (HL) and non-Hodgkin lymphoma (NHL) may present as an anterior mediastinal mass.
- The presence and distribution of mediastinal disease is important for both staging purposes and treatment planning.
- Even though NHLs account for more than 80% of all cases of lymphoma and roughly half of affected patients have intrathoracic disease at the time of diagnosis, HL is approximately three times more common in the mediastinum than NHL.
- Diffuse large B-cell lymphoma is an aggressive form of NHL and the most common type of lymphoma.
- One-third of patients present with systemic manifestations ("B" symptoms), such as fever, night sweats, weight loss, malaise, and fatigue.

- HL commonly presents as mediastinal lymphadenopathy, with the anterior mediastinum and right paratracheal lymph nodes more commonly involved.
- HL more commonly presents as a mediastinal mass with homogeneous density.
- Large lymphomas, both HLs and NHLs, may present with heterogeneous density as a result of hemorrhage and necrosis.
- Occasionally (5%), calcification may be seen in thoracic lymphomas at the time of diagnosis. Extensive dystrophic calcification is more common following radiation therapy.
- Mediastinal lymphoma is, after lung cancer, the second most common tumoral cause of superior vena cava syndrome.
- Fluorodeoxyglucose positron emission tomography (PET) provides whole-body images for the initial staging and later follow-up of patients with lymphoma.

✓ Pearls & ✗ Pitfalls

- ✓ Parenchymal pulmonary involvement may be seen both in HL and in NHL.
- ✗ The evaluation of lymph node involvement by CT, based mainly on size criteria, is limited. Lymph nodes with a normal size may be involved. PET better defines abnormal lymph nodes by demonstrating increased metabolic activity. Additionally, a lymph node may be enlarged without having tumoral involvement.

Case 22

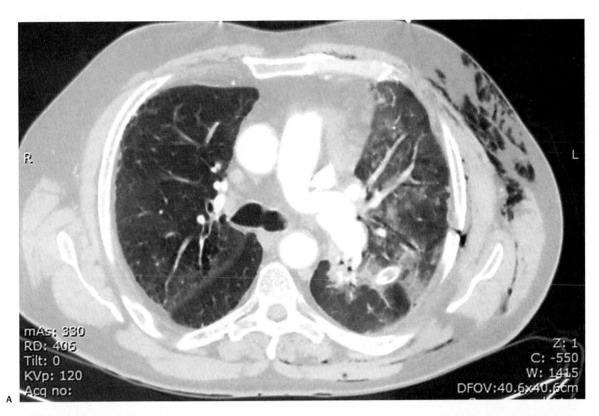

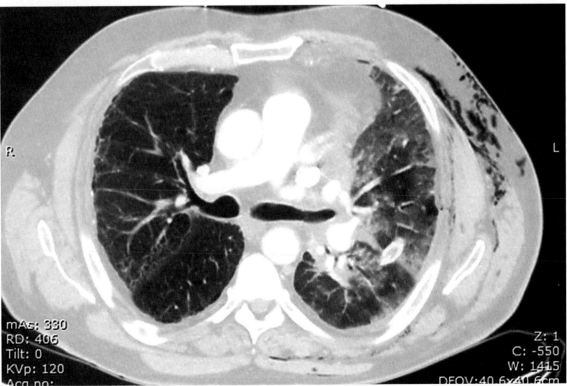

▪ Clinical Presentation

An adult man in whom severe respiratory distress developed 36 hours after he received a left lung transplant.

■ Imaging Findings

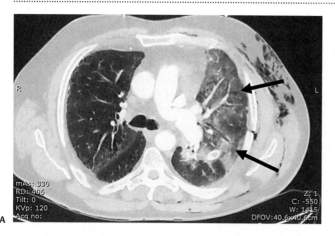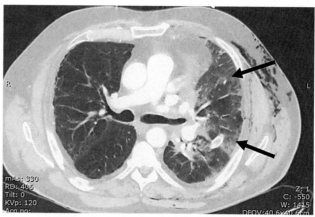

(A,B) Computed tomography of the chest demonstrates extensive ground-glass parenchymal opacity diffusely involving the newly transplanted left lung (*arrows*). Postoperative left-sided subcutaneous emphysema is also present.

■ Differential Diagnosis

- ***Reperfusion pulmonary edema:*** Reperfusion edema, also known as reimplantation response, is a form of noncardiogenic pulmonary edema commonly seen in the first 2 or 3 days after lung transplant and should be suspected when ground-glass opacities develop in the early postoperative period.
- *Acute rejection:* Parenchymal disease with the development of ground-glass opacities and consolidation around the second week after lung transplant is concerning for acute rejection.
- *Pneumonia:* Infection is probably the most common complication after lung transplant and can be seen both early and late after the transplant. Bacterial, viral, and fungal pneumonias may present with a variable degree of air-space consolidation. Cytomegalovirus and *Pseudomonas* are the two infectious organisms most commonly responsible for pneumonias in the first 2 months.

■ Essential Facts

- Reimplantation response, also known as reperfusion edema, is a common abnormality seen to some extent in the majority (> 95%) of patients after lung transplant.
- This is a form of noncardiogenic pulmonary edema.
- It usually starts around postoperative day 1, peaks around day 5, and resolves around day 8.

- Reperfusion pulmonary edema should not extend beyond the first postoperative week.
- There is a clear association between the severity of reperfusion edema and the ischemic time of the graft.
- The pathophysiology is multifactorial, with surgical trauma, capillary ischemia, interruption of the lymphatic drainage and bronchial circulation, and surfactant deficiency contributing to an increase in capillary permeability.
- Reperfusion edema typically starts as perihilar opacities, with peribronchial and perivascular edema and indistinctness.
- Treatment usually consists of mechanical ventilatory support and diuresis.
- As in other forms of edema, interlobular septal thickening and ground-glass opacities that may progress to air-space consolidation are common findings.

✓ Pearls & ✗ Pitfalls

- ✓ Reimplantation response that extends beyond postoperative day 10 raises concern for acute rejection or pulmonary infection.
- ✗ Reperfusion pulmonary edema can very easily be mistaken for cardiogenic pulmonary edema. In the case of a patient with a single lung transplant, the unilateral distribution favors reimplantation response. In a patient with a bilateral lung transplant, if the reimplantation response affects both lungs, the differentiation is more difficult.

Case 23

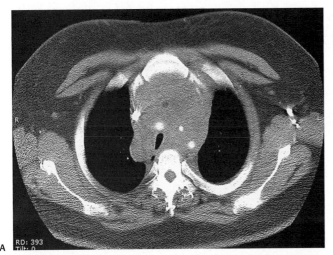

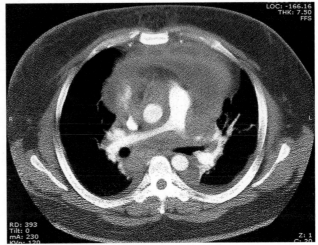

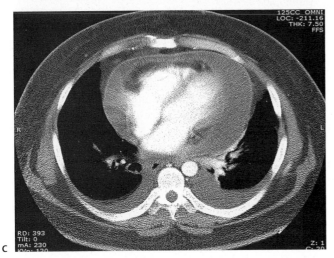

■ Clinical Presentation

Fatigue, anemia, petechiae, and easy bruising in a 24-year-old man.

■ Imaging Findings

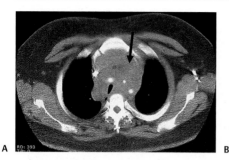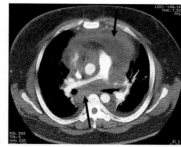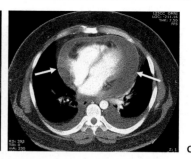

(A–C) Contrast-enhanced computed tomography of the chest shows a large mediastinal mass diffusely infiltrating the different compartments of the mediastinum (*black arrows*). Pericardial involvement (*white arrows*) as well as bilateral pleural fluid collections are also noted.

■ Differential Diagnosis

- ***Leukemia (acute lymphocytic leukemia [ALL]):*** Abnormally enlarged mediastinal lymph nodes or diffuse mediastinal masses are commonly seen in acute and chronic leukemias.
- *Lymphoma:* Both Hodgkin and non-Hodgkin lymphomas may present with extensive mediastinal involvement, as well as pleural and pericardial effusion.
- *Small-cell lung cancer:* An extensive mediastinal mass may be seen at the initial presentation or during the course of disease in small-cell lung cancer.

■ Essential Facts

- Four major types of leukemia are recognized, depending on type of cell (myelogenous or lymphocytic) and type of clinical presentation and evolution (acute or chronic): ALL, chronic lymphocytic leukemia (CLL), acute myelogenous leukemia, and chronic myelogenous leukemia.
- Nearly 45,000 new cases of leukemia are diagnosed each year in the United States.
- Most cases of leukemia present in adults (average age at diagnosis of 67 years); leukemia is 10 times more common in adults than in children.
- CLL is the most common type of leukemia in adults, whereas ALL is the most common type in children.
- Generalized lymphadenopathy is a common finding in some types of leukemia (e.g., adult T-cell leukemia, ALL, and CLL) and is seen in more than 50% of cases in some series.
- Pleural effusion or plaquelike pleural thickening is reported in as many as one-third of patients with leukemia in autopsy series but is less commonly seen in these patients clinically (10%).

- The frequency of respiratory involvement in patients with acute leukemia is high. Respiratory involvement results either from pulmonary infiltration by leukemia or from pulmonary hemorrhage.
- The most common imaging findings in the lung parenchyma are ground-glass attenuation, centrilobular nodules, and interlobular septal thickening.
- Patients with leukemia who have undergone bone marrow transplant may also present with pulmonary complications, such as bacterial pneumonia or opportunistic infections (e.g., *Pneumocystis* pneumonia, cytomegalovirus infection, *Aspergillus* infection).
- More than 60% of deaths in patients with leukemia are due to infectious disease, which tends to occur after chemotherapy or in the neutropenic stage after bone marrow transplant.
- Granulocytic sarcomas or chloromas are tumors formed by immature granulocytes, derived from myeloid cell precursors, that can be seen in acute myelocytic leukemia or ALL. The most common locations in the thorax are in the subperiosteal region of the ribs or sternum, or in relation to the thoracic vertebral bodies. Occasionally, these tumors may also be seen in the soft tissues or skin.

✓ Pearls & ✗ Pitfalls

- ✓ In the majority of patients with leukemic pulmonary infiltrates, pulmonary disease is strongly associated with an elevated number of blast cells (peripheral blast count > 40%).
- ✗ Thoracic imaging findings in patients with leukemia are nonspecific. In particular, the imaging findings in the lung parenchyma may represent leukemic infiltration, drug toxicity, pulmonary edema, or infection.

Case 24

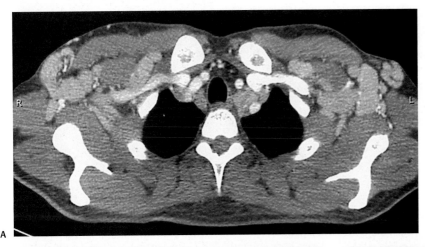

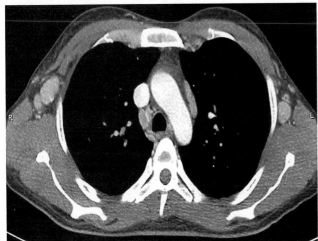

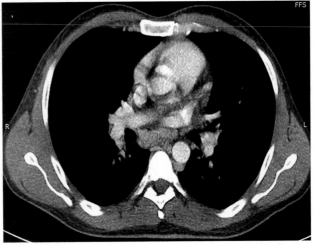

■ Clinical Presentation

A man positive for human immunodeficiency virus presenting with fever and weight loss.

■ Imaging Findings

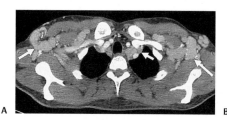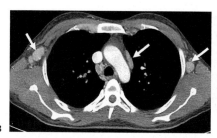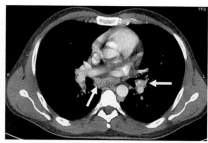

(A–C) Contrast-enhanced computed tomography (CT) of the thorax demonstrates multiple enhancing lymph nodes bilaterally in the axillae, mediastinum, and pulmonary hila (*arrows*).

■ Differential Diagnosis

- ***Multicentric Castleman disease (MCD):*** Multifocal hypervascular lymphadenopathy is characteristic of MCD.
- *Kaposi sarcoma:* Hypervascular lymphadenopathy may be seen in Kaposi sarcoma, which is also an important entity to be considered in the differential diagnosis of human immunodeficiency virus (HIV)-infected individuals with enhancing lymph nodes.
- *Lymphoma:* The generalized lymphadenopathy seen in HIV-infected patients may be secondary to lymphoma or may be reactive lymphadenopathy (follicular hyperplasia), but it is usually without significant enhancement on contrast CT.

■ Essential Facts

- Generalized or MCD is characterized by the simultaneous involvement of different anatomic sites.
- Castleman disease in HIV-infected patients is typically multicentric (MCD), has a more aggressive clinical course than the localized form, and is associated with a high mortality rate (> 60%).
- In the HIV population, MCD, like Kaposi sarcoma, is mediated by human herpesvirus type 8 (HHV8), which explains why a large number of these patients (> 70%) have both conditions.
- The plasma cell variant is the characteristic histologic type in more than 90% of cases of MCD.

- Systemic symptoms, including fever, weight loss, cough, and dyspnea, are common.
- Enlarged lymph nodes are commonly seen in the mediastinum, axillae, retrocrural space, celiac trunk, paraortic, and inguinal regions.
- Anemia and a low CD4-cell count are common abnormal laboratory findings.
- Other complications that have been reported in HIV-positive patients with MCD are multiple pulmonary nodules, interstitial pneumonitis, pleural effusion, respiratory distress syndrome, and non-Hodgkin lymphoma.
- Splenomegaly (100%) and hepatomegaly (85%) are common imaging and clinical findings in patients with MCD.

✓ Pearls & ✗ Pitfalls

✓ It is common for clinical symptoms to wax and wane in HIV-related cases of MCD. Episodes of exacerbation, or "attacks," coincide with an increase in the viral loads of HHV8 in the peripheral blood and bronchoalveolar lavage specimens.

✗ Non–contrast-enhanced examinations are less sensitive than contrast-enhanced examinations to detect the characteristic hypervascular nature of the lymph nodes seen in patients with MCD.

Case 25

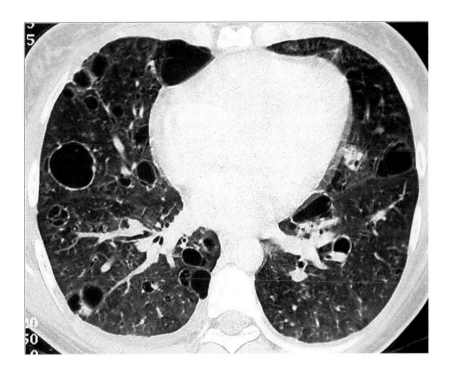

■ Clinical Presentation

A 46-year-old woman with Sjögren syndrome.

■ Imaging Findings

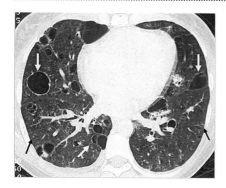

Thoracic computed tomography lung window image demonstrates a thin-walled cyst as well as small nodules (*white arrows*) and minimal interlobular septal thickening in both lungs (*black arrows*).

■ Differential Diagnosis

- ***Lymphocytic interstitial pneumonia (LIP):*** In the clinical setting of a patient with Sjögren syndrome, the presence of small, thin-walled pulmonary cysts is consistent with LIP.
- Pneumocystis jiroveci *infection:* Cystic changes with thin-walled cysts, nodules, and ground-glass opacities are common findings in *Pneumocystis* infection.
- *Langerhans cell histiocytosis and lymphangioleiomyomatosis:* These two conditions may manifest as cystic changes in the lungs, are also associated with pulmonary nodules, and should be considered in the differential diagnosis of cystic lung lesions.

■ Essential Facts

- LIP is a lymphoproliferative condition in which the lungs are diffusely infiltrated with benign lymphoid elements.
- LIP is characterized by a diffuse interstitial proliferation of lymphocytes and plasma cells involving the interlobular and alveolar septa.
- The most commonly affected individuals are middle-aged women who have systemic diseases associated with some form of immunologic dysfunction.
- Among the concurrent conditions, Sjögren syndrome is the most common, followed by autoimmune thyroiditis and systemic lupus erythematosus.
- Other conditions associated with LIP include active hepatitis, primary biliary cirrhosis, myasthenia gravis, Castleman disease, rheumatoid arthritis, pernicious anemia, and autoimmune hemolytic anemia.

- A clear association between human immunodeficiency virus (HIV) infection and LIP exists in the pediatric population, and LIP in children is considered to be an acquired immunodeficiency syndrome–defining illness.
- Other immunodeficiency conditions, such as agammaglobulinemia, hypogammaglobulinemia, and common variable immunodeficiency, have also been associated with LIP.
- Patients with LIP are usually symptomatic with dyspnea and cough.
- Imaging findings consist of ground-glass opacities, centrilobular nodules, bronchovascular bundle thickening, and pulmonary cysts.
- The lower lobes are more significantly involved.
- Mediastinal and hilar lymph node enlargement is a relatively common imaging finding in LIP.

✓ Pearls & ✗ Pitfalls

- ✓ Several studies have linked the development of LIP to viral infections, mainly with HIV, Epstein-Barr virus, and human T-lymphotropic virus.
- ✗ Some of the imaging findings described in LIP, including bronchovascular bundle thickening, patchy consolidation, ground-glass opacities, and subpleural nodules, are nonspecific and may be seen in other lymphoproliferative lung disorders, such as pulmonary lymphoma.

Case 26

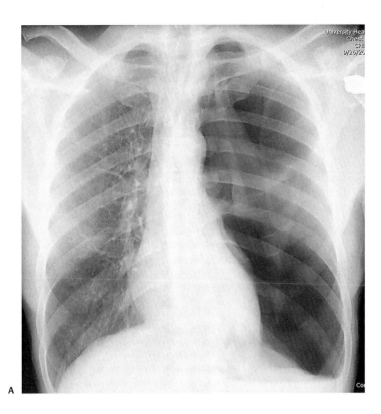

A

Clinical Presentation

Before and after placement of a left-sided thoracostomy tube in a patient with left-sided pneumothorax. The patient had left-sided chest pain for the previous 3 days.

Further Work-up

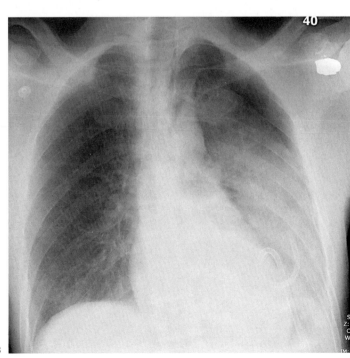

B

■ Imaging Findings

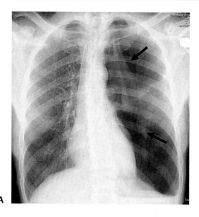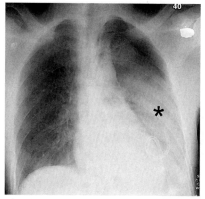

(A) Initial chest radiograph demonstrates a large left-sided pneumothorax (*arrows*). **(B)** After placement of a thoracostomy tube, radiograph shows significant re-expansion of the left lung with interval development of diffuse parenchymal opacities in the same lung (*asterisk*).

■ Differential Diagnosis

- ***Re-expansion pulmonary edema (RPE):*** The development of diffuse pulmonary parenchymal opacities after re-expansion of a lung collapsed from pneumothorax or drainage of a large pleural effusion is consistent with RPE.
- *Pulmonary contusion:* In trauma patients with unilateral posttraumatic pneumothorax, ipsilateral or bilateral parenchymal opacity may result from pulmonary contusion.
- Pneumocystis *pneumonia:* Diffuse unilateral parenchymal opacity may represent pneumonia. Infections with agents such as *Pneumocystis jiroveci* may present with spontaneous pneumothorax resulting from the rupture of pulmonary cysts.

■ Essential Facts

- RPE was first described after the rapid drainage of large pleural effusions.
- Later, RPE after re-expansion of a lung collapsed from pneumothorax was also described.
- Possible mechanisms for the development of RPE have been postulated: a reduction in surfactant production; a combination of factors, including a rapid increase in blood flow to the lung during re-expansion in which the abrupt increase in capillary pressure leads to liquid and protein overflow to the lung interstitium and air space.

- Currently, two major mechanisms are considered responsible: an alteration of capillary permeability and an increase in hydrostatic pressure.
- More than 80% of cases of RPE occur in patients with prolonged pulmonary collapse (> 72 hours).
- The speed of pulmonary re-expansion is more significant than the use of negative pressure in the development of RPE.
- Inflammatory mediators (polymorphonuclear cells, interleukin-8, and monocyte chemotactic protein) are additional factors in the development of RPE.
- In ~7% of cases, the pulmonary edema is bilateral.
- Imaging findings in RPE vary from interstitial edema with the presence of Kerley B lines to alveolar edema with airspace consolidation.

✓ Pearls & ✗ Pitfalls

- ✓ In at least in one published series, the mortality rate associated with RPE was high (> 20%), which highlights the seriousness of this condition.
- ✗ Cardiogenic pulmonary edema may be unilateral. The distribution of cardiogenic (hydrostatic) pulmonary edema is typically bilateral, but occasionally unilateral distribution may occur. Other causes of unilateral pulmonary edema include contralateral pulmonary embolism, pulmonary vein stenosis, and mitral valve regurgitation.

Case 27

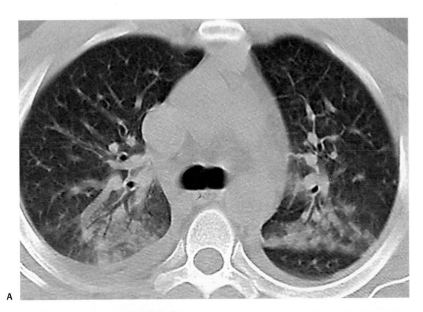

A

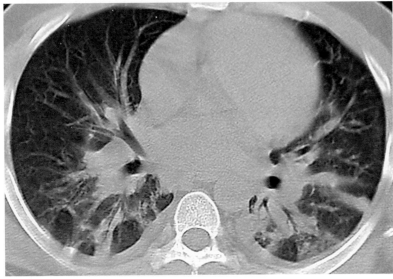

B

■ Clinical Presentation

A 30-year-old man with progressive shortness of breath after a heroin binge.

■ Imaging Findings

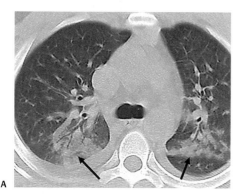 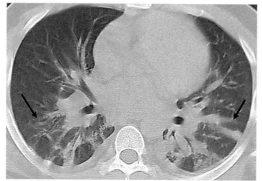

A   B

(A,B) Computed tomography of the chest demonstrates bilateral parenchymal opacities with air-space consolidation in the basilar and dependent aspects of the lungs (*arrows*). Small pleural effusions are also appreciated bilaterally.

■ Differential Diagnosis

- **Heroin-induced pulmonary edema:** Bilateral parenchymal opacities in a patient with a history of heroin overdose are a common presentation of heroin-induced pulmonary edema.
- *Pneumonia:* Drug abusers are at increased risk for human immunodeficiency virus infection and for the development of community-acquired pneumonia and opportunistic infections, which may present with a multifocal and bilateral distribution.
- *Aspiration:* The altered mental status of a patient with heroin overdose is associated with an increased risk for aspiration.

■ Essential Facts

- Heroin use and heroin-related visits to the emergency department have increased dramatically in the United States.
- The typical patient is a young man.
- Heroin overdose is a serious condition with significant mortality.
- Pulmonary edema develops in a minority of patients with heroin overdose (2%), but pulmonary edema is commonly seen in those who die.
- Altered mental status, pinpoint pupils, and severely decreased respiratory drive are a common clinical triad in cases of heroin overdose.

- The initial management of these patients includes the administration of naloxone and oxygen supplementation.
- Pulmonary edema secondary to heroin overdose should be suspected if there is persistent hypoxia after the respiratory rate has normalized and if fluffy alveolar opacities are seen on chest radiographs.
- The majority of these respiratory symptoms resolve within 24 hours.
- As many as one-third of these patients eventually require intubation and mechanical ventilation.
- Imaging findings consist of bilateral parenchymal opacities in the majority of patients.
- Increased capillary permeability, not heart failure, is considered to be the cause of heroin-induced pulmonary edema.
- Patchy atelectasis and nodular opacities may also be seen in patients with heroin-induced pulmonary edema.

✓ Pearls & ✗ Pitfalls

- ✓ Approximately half of patients presenting to the emergency department with heroin overdose test positive for cocaine and/or alcohol. Cocaine is known to produce both cardiogenic and noncardiogenic pulmonary edema.
- ✗ As many as one-fourth of patients who have heroin-induced pulmonary edema present with unilateral disease on imaging examinations.

Case 28

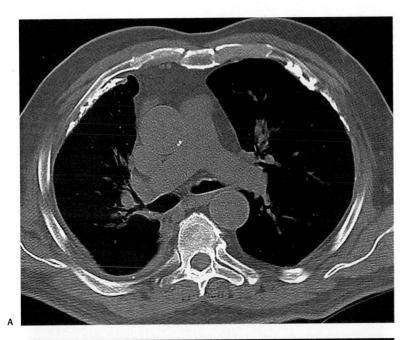

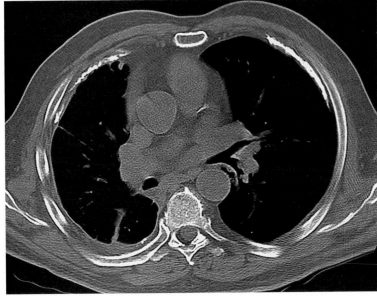

■ Clinical Presentation

A 55-year-old man with progressive shortness of breath who has abnormal findings on chest radiography.

■ Imaging Findings

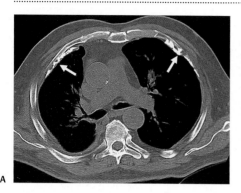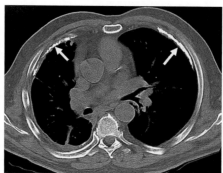

(A,B) Non–contrast-enhanced computed tomography (CT) of the chest shows pleural thickening and extensively calcified pleural plaques bilaterally (*arrows*).

■ Differential Diagnosis

- ***Asbestos-related pleural plaques:*** Bilateral calcified pleural plaques are a characteristic presentation of asbestos-related pleural disease.
- *Postinfectious pleural plaques:* Chronic infection, such as pulmonary tuberculosis, can also present with pleural thickening and calcified plaques. The pattern is usually unilateral and relatively diffuse, whereas the pattern seen in asbestos exposure is bilateral and focal.
- *Posthemorrhagic pleural thickening:* Hemothorax may also produce pleural thickening that can calcify in the long run. This is also more commonly a unilateral finding.

■ Essential Facts

- Asbestos-related pleural disease includes pleural effusion, pleural plaques, pleural thickening, and malignant mesothelioma.
- Pleural disease is the most common clinical and imaging manifestation of asbestos exposure.
- The earliest manifestation of pleural disease after asbestos exposure is pleural effusion, which is typically hemorrhagic and usually presents approximately 10 years after the exposure.
- Pleural plaques, which are focal, discrete areas of fibrosis that usually arise from the parietal pleura, are the most common manifestation of asbestos exposure.

- These plaques tend to occur later, 20 or 30 years after chronic asbestos exposure. They are commonly bilateral, involve the mid and lower pleural surfaces, and calcify in about 15% of cases.
- On histologic examination, these plaques are seen to be composed mainly of acellular collagen with visible asbestos fibers.
- Diffuse pleural thickening, another manifestation of asbestos exposure, is less specific than pleural plaques and can result from multiple exudative and inflammatory processes.
- When pleural plaques involve the visceral pleura, short linear densities (hairy plaques) radiate from the plaques to the adjacent lung parenchyma.

✓ Pearls & ✗ Pitfalls

- ✓ Bilateral pleural plaques on the diaphragmatic surface are considered almost pathognomonic for asbestos exposure.
- ✗ Extrapleural fat and rib fractures may mimic asbestos-related pleural plaques on conventional radiographs. CT is more sensitive (97% vs. 60%) and more specific for the visualization and characterization of asbestos-related pleural disease.

Case 29

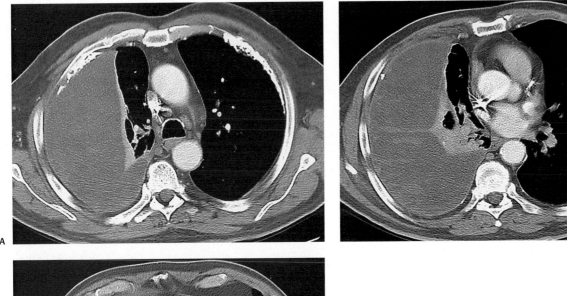

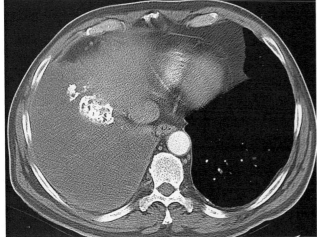

■ Clinical Presentation

A 74-year-old man with right-sided chest pain and weight loss.

■ Imaging Findings

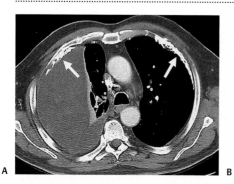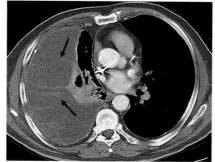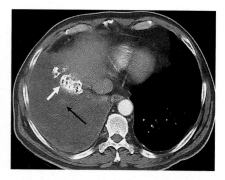

A   B   C

(A–C) Contrast-enhanced computed tomography of the chest shows a large right-sided pleural opacity with ill-defined linear areas of enhancement (*black arrows*), as well as densely calcified pleural plaques bilaterally, including a calcified plaque on the right diaphragmatic surface (*white arrows*).

■ Differential Diagnosis

- ***Malignant pleural mesothelioma (MPM):*** Enhancing tissue and calcified pleural plaques are suggestive of asbestos-related pleural mesothelioma.
- *Loculated empyema:* Chronic infection within the pleural space may be associated with significant pleural thickening, fluid, and enhancing septa.
- *Adenocarcinoma:* Pleural involvement from a metastatic tumor, in particular adenocarcinoma, may present as a mixture of pleural thickening, enhancing tissue, and pleural fluid.

■ Essential Facts

- The most common primary tumor of the pleura is malignant mesothelioma, which has a strong association with exposure to asbestos, in particular to crocidolite, or blue asbestos.
- A long period of latency is required for the development of malignant mesothelioma after exposure to asbestos, typically more than 20 years.
- The most common histologic subtypes are the epithelial (50%), sarcomatous (20%), and mixed (biphasic) types (30%).
- A dose-dependent relationship exists; the lifetime risk for the development of MPM in any asbestos worker is 10%.
- Persons at risk include not only occupationally exposed workers but also members of their household and persons residing near asbestos mines and industrial plants that process these fibers.
- The tumor may arise from either the visceral or the parietal pleura, commonly presenting with associated pleural effusion.
- MPM has a poor prognosis, with few patients surviving more than 1 year after diagnosis.
- Initial spread involves the pleural surface and pericardium, with later lymphangitis and hematogenous dissemination to distant organs (lungs, liver, kidneys).
- Imaging findings include unilateral nodular or smooth pleural thickening, effusion, and tissue infiltration of the interlobar pulmonary fissures, which results in circumferential growth and entrapment of the lung with associated volume loss.
- Calcified pleural plaques consistent with asbestos-related pleural disease may be seen in 20 to 50% of patients with malignant mesothelioma.

✓ Pearls & ✗ Pitfalls

- ✓ MPM is a locally aggressive tumor that may invade the chest wall, diaphragm, and mediastinum.
- ✗ The differentiation between MPM and metastatic adenocarcinoma is difficult. The imaging and light microscopy appearances of these two tumors are similar. Immunohistochemical techniques are usually required to differentiate the two entities.

Case 30

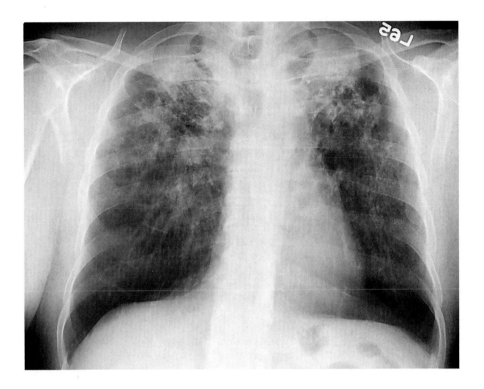

■ Clinical Presentation

A 59-year-old miner with progressive dyspnea on exertion.

■ Imaging Findings

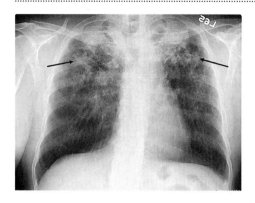

Conventional chest radiograph reveals extensive areas of confluent and masslike fibronodular opacities in both upper lobes, with calcification and apical pleural thickening (*arrows*). There is upper lobe volume loss bilaterally, with cephalic retraction of the pulmonary hila. An area of lucency is seen in the left upper lobe.

■ Differential Diagnosis

- *Silicosis:* Complicated silicosis (progressive massive fibrosis) is characterized by masslike opacities resulting from the coalescence of fibronodular fibrosis. It tends to affect the upper lobes more often.
- *Tuberculosis (TB):* Bilateral apical fibronodular opacities with apical pleural thickening and upper lobe volume loss in particular are associated with cavitation and may be sequelae of chronic reactivation TB or atypical mycobacterial infection.
- *Sarcoidosis:* In a subset of patients with sarcoidosis (20%), the dominant pattern is the development of massive fibrosis, predominantly in the upper lobes.

■ Essential Facts

- Silicosis, the most prevalent pneumoconiosis, is an occupational disease that results from the chronic aspiration of free crystalline silica dust, a major component of the earth's crust.
- Silicone dioxide, in the form of small particles that deposit in the respiratory bronchioles, is the chemical compound responsible for inducing the inflammatory reaction in the lung parenchyma.
- Occupations such as mining, tunneling, quarrying, sandblasting, polishing, and stonecutting are the ones most commonly associated with this condition.
- The most commonly affected regions are the upper lobes and the superior segment of the lower lobes bilaterally.
- Simple silicosis is characterized by the presence of multiple small (1–10 mm), well-defined pulmonary nodules, uniform in shape and mainly peripheral in distribution.
- A centrilobular distribution, predominantly on the posterior aspect of the lungs, has been noted on computed tomographic examination.

- Calcification of these small nodules is seen in fewer than 20% of cases.
- Complicated silicosis, also known as progressive massive fibrosis, is characterized by confluent nodules forming opacities > 1 cm in diameter and an increased amount of fibrosis, occasionally with dystrophic calcification and cavitation.
- Eggshell calcification of hilar and mediastinal lymph nodes is a common finding in patients with silicosis.
- Acute silicosis, or silicoproteinosis, is a rare form of the disease associated with massive exposure to silica dust, usually in enclosed spaces. It develops after a relatively short exposure (usually months), progresses rapidly, and has a poor prognosis.
- Foci of irregular (cicatricial) emphysema are often seen adjacent to the areas of confluent fibrosis in patients with complicated silicosis.

✓ Pearls & ✗ Pitfalls

✓ Caplan syndrome, also known as rheumatoid pneumoconiosis, is a rare variant of silicosis, coal worker pneumoconiosis, and other pneumoconioses that is seen in patients with rheumatoid disease and lung involvement. It is characterized by large necrobiotic nodules superimposed on a background of multiple pulmonary nodules.

✗ Coal worker pneumoconiosis results from the aspiration of a mixture of inorganic dusts, including coal, mica, kaolin, and silica, and is not the same condition as silicosis. The two entities have a different clinical course; in coal worker pneumoconiosis, there is significantly less fibrosis. However, the imaging presentations may be similar, with innumerable small pulmonary nodules.

Case 31

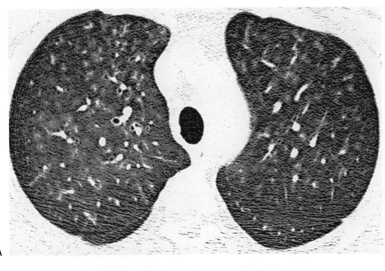

A

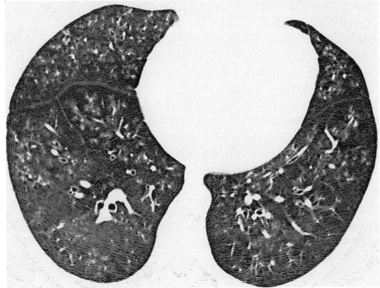

B

▪ Clinical Presentation

A young adult woodworker with recurrent "asthma" attacks that begin while he is working. The respiratory symptoms abate if he stays at home.

■ Imaging Findings

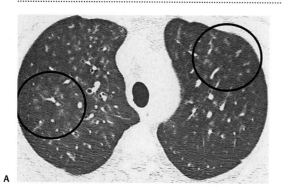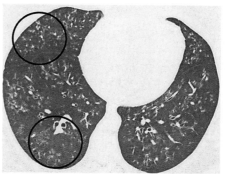

A   B

(A,B) Computed tomography (CT) of the chest reveals ground-glass centrilobular nodules and a mild degree of bronchial wall thickening in a multilobar distribution. In some areas, more diffuse ground-glass opacity is appreciated (*circles*).

■ Differential Diagnosis

- **Hypersensitivity pneumonitis (HP):** Centrilobular ground-glass nodules and patchy areas of ground-glass opacity are commonly seen in HP.
- *Atypical infection:* Viral infection and infection with *Mycoplasma* or *Chlamydia* may present as ground-glass centrilobular nodules and patchy ground-glass opacities.
- *Diffuse alveolar hemorrhage:* Goodpasture syndrome and different forms of vasculitis may present with diffuse alveolar hemorrhage that manifests as ground-glass nodules and opacities.

■ Essential Facts

- HP, or extrinsic allergic alveolitis, is a complex and heterogeneous group of disorders that result from the inhalation of various airborne organic particles.
- In a susceptible host, the particles induce an immune-mediated reaction in the airways and pulmonary parenchyma.
- Causative particles may be bacteria, fungi, avian proteins, wood dusts, and certain chemical compounds.
- Histopathologic features of HP include neutrophilic infiltration, cellular bronchiolitis, lymphocytic infiltrates, small, noncaseating granulomas, and areas of organizing pneumonia.
- In a large number of cases, the offending agent is never identified.
- The clinical presentation includes fever, chills, dyspnea, cough, weight loss, and fatigue.

- Three major clinical forms of HP are recognized: acute, subacute, and chronic.
- Recurrent subacute episodes of HP may lead to pulmonary fibrosis.
- Typical findings in the acute phase are centrilobular ground-glass nodules and ground-glass patchy opacities.
- The middle and lower lung zones may be more significantly affected.
- Chronic exposure to the antigen can result in interstitial pulmonary fibrosis with reticulation, traction bronchiectasis, and some degree of honeycombing, resembling nonspecific interstitial pneumonia.
- The finding of fibrosis on CT is associated with increased mortality and a poor prognosis.
- Air trapping on expiratory high-resolution CT (HRCT) may also be seen and reflects the presence of respiratory bronchiolitis, a common histopathologic feature in HP.

✓ Pearls & ✗ Pitfalls

✓ The best-known forms of hypersensitivity pneumonitis include farmer lung, bird fancier lung, bagassosis, and hot tub lung.

✗ During acute and subacute episodes of HP, findings on conventional chest radiographs are commonly normal. A significant number of symptomatic patients with normal chest radiographic findings will have abnormal findings on HRCT.

Case 32

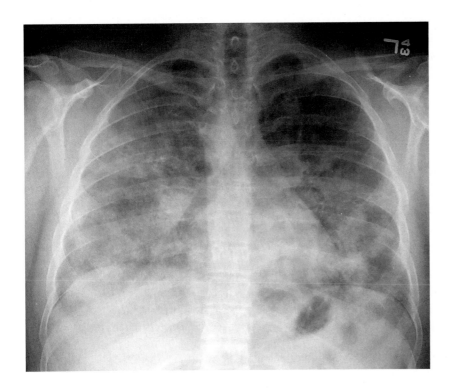

■ Clinical Presentation

A 34-year-old man with chronic cough.

■ **Imaging Findings**

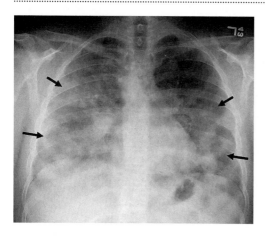

Chest radiograph shows dense, multifocal parenchymal ground-glass opacities and denser areas of consolidation that are more confluent in the mid and lower lung zones. There is relative sparing of the apices (*arrows*). There is no evidence of pleural fluid, and the cardiac silhouette is normal in size. Incidental note is made of a right-sided aortic arch.

■ **Differential Diagnosis**

- ***Pulmonary alveolar proteinosis (PAP):*** Ground-glass opacity with air-space consolidation in a bilateral and multifocal distribution is a common imaging presentation of PAP.
- *Pulmonary edema:* Pulmonary edema may also present with interlobular septal thickening, ground-glass opacification, and even air-space consolidation.
- *Atypical pneumonia:* Viral pneumonia, *Mycoplasma* infection, *Chlamydia* infection, and *Pneumocystis jiroveci* pneumonia may also present with a mixture of ground-glass opacity and interlobular septal thickening in a bilateral multilobar distribution.

■ **Essential Facts**

- PAP is an uncommon condition characterized by the abnormal accumulation of lipoproteinaceous material in the pulmonary alveoli.
- This granular eosinophilic material corresponds to pulmonary surfactant, which accumulates because of reduced clearance, not because of increased production.
- Affected patients have an increased susceptibility to pulmonary and extrapulmonary infection from both common and opportunistic organisms.
- Three distinct clinical forms of the disease are known: congenital, idiopathic (acquired), and secondary.
- The congenital form is rare (< 2% of cases), is seen in neonates, and has a poor prognosis.
- The secondary form (8%) has been described in association with cancer, human immunodeficiency virus infection,

silicosis, and the aspiration of different chemicals and particles that lead to a reduced number or impaired function of alveolar macrophages.
- The idiopathic form (90%) most commonly affects men about 40 years of age with a history of cigarette smoking (> 70%).
- Clinical manifestations include cough, dyspnea, fever, hemoptysis, and chest pain.
- The natural history of PAP is variable; in a small proportion of patients, it resolves spontaneously. The majority of patients either have stable but persistent disease or experience progressive respiratory deterioration.
- The 5-year survival rate after the diagnosis is > 75%.
- Typical imaging findings on conventional chest radiographs consist of bilateral air-space disease that is more confluent in the mid lung zones and parahilar regions, similar to the "bat wing" distribution seen in pulmonary edema.
- On plain films, PAP generally spares the lung apices and lateral costophrenic angles.

✓ **Pearls & ✗ Pitfalls**

✓ Acquired or idiopathic PAP is most likely an autoimmune disease targeting granulocyte-macrophage colony-stimulating-factor.

✗ The imaging findings of PAP and cardiogenic pulmonary edema on plain films are similar. The absence of plural effusion and a normal cardiac silhouette favor the diagnosis of PAP.

Case 33

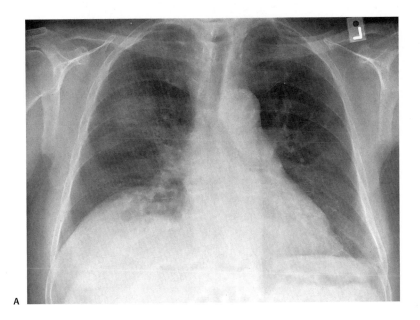

Clinical Presentation

A 61-year-old man with cough. His past medical history is remarkable only for chronic constipation.

Further Work-up

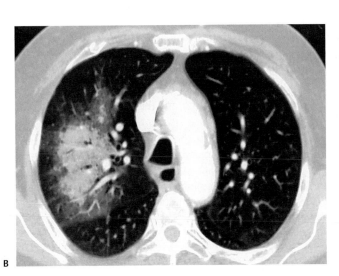

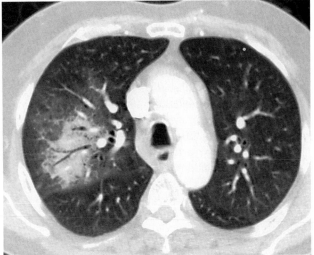

■ Imaging Findings

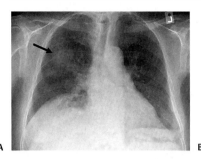 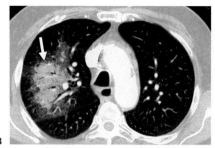 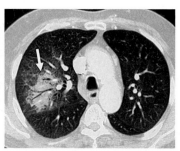

A   B   C

(A) Chest radiograph reveals an ill-defined area of parenchymal consolidation in the right upper lobe (*arrow*). **(B,C)** Computed tomography (CT) of the chest with two different window levels; within the area of denser opacity, subtle focal hypodensities are noted (*arrows*).

■ Differential Diagnosis

- ***Exogenous lipoid pneumonia:*** Radiographs and CT scans of the chest in patients with exogenous lipoid pneumonia characteristically reveal air-space consolidation and masslike opacity, occasionally with areas of low attenuation.
- *Pneumonia:* Community-acquired pneumonia is the most common cause of a focal area of air-space consolidation in a segmental, lobar, or multifocal distribution.
- *Lung cancer:* Certain types of lung cancer, like bronchioloalveolar carcinoma, may present with air-space consolidation, mimicking pneumonia.

■ Essential Facts

- Lipoid pneumonia can be classified as exogenous or endogenous, depending on the source and origin of the intra-alveolar lipid.
- Exogenous lipoid pneumonia results from the acute or chronic aspiration or inhalation of oily substances like mineral oil, vegetable oil, and animal oil into the air spaces.
- Mineral oil is relatively inert and ingested by macrophages, and when chronically aspirated, it may induce a foreign body inflammatory reaction, with fibrosis and the formation of a mass (paraffinoma).
- The most common cause of exogenous lipoid pneumonia in the elderly is the aspiration of mineral oil used as a laxative. The next most common cause is the inhalation of mineral oil nose drops used for chronic rhinitis.

- The most common distribution is controversial. Classic reports have mentioned a higher prevalence in the right lung in the dependent aspect of the affected lobes: the posterior segment of the lower lobes or the posterior segment of an upper lobe. Recently, in a series of cases, a bilateral distribution was the most commonly observed pattern.
- The treatment of exogenous lipoid pneumonia basically consists of preventing additional exposure.
- Follow-up examination reveals slow regression or a stable appearance of the abnormality.
- Endogenous lipoid pneumonia results from the degeneration of alveolar cell walls distal to an airway obstruction, usually from a lung cancer.
- A crazy-paving pattern on thin-slice CT has been also described in patients with exogenous lipoid pneumonia.

✓ Pearls & ✗ Pitfalls

- ✓ The diagnosis of exogenous lipoid pneumonia is based on the history of exposure, the presence of an opacity on imaging examination, and the presence of lipid-laden macrophages in bronchoalveolar lavage or lung biopsy specimens.
- ✗ A consolidation or masslike irregular opacity with low density on CT (–30 to –120 Hounsfield units) is highly suggestive of intrapulmonary fat and lipoid pneumonia. The prevalence of this finding is variable, reported in 15 to 70% of patients with exogenous lipoid pneumonia.

Case 34

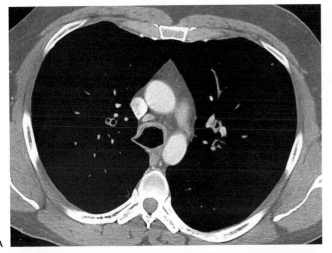

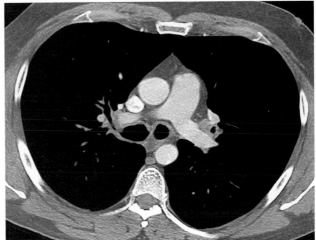

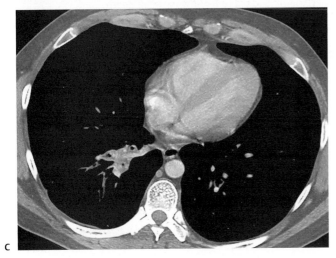

▇ Clinical Presentation

A 42-year-old man with cough, hoarseness, and throat pain.

■ Imaging Findings

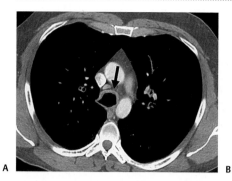 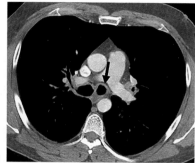 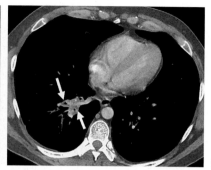

(A–C) Contrast-enhanced computed tomography (CT) of the chest: axial images at three different levels show abnormal thickening of the anterior and lateral tracheal wall (*black arrows*) as well as right lower lobe concentric bronchial wall thickening and luminal narrowing (*white arrows*).

■ Differential Diagnosis

- **Relapsing polychondritis:** Anterior and lateral tracheal wall thickening that spares the posterior membranous portion and concentric bronchial wall thickening are characteristic findings of relapsing polychondritis.
- *Amyloidosis/sarcoidosis:* Airway involvement in amyloidosis and sarcoidosis may manifest as airway thickening with a variable degree of stenosis.
- *Tracheopathia osteochondroplastica:* Nodular tracheal wall thickening, usually with calcification, is the typical presentation of tracheopathia osteochondroplastica.

■ Essential Facts

- Relapsing polychondritis is a rare, chronic, multisystem autoimmune inflammatory disorder characterized by recurrent episodes of inflammation and destruction of cartilaginous tissue.
- All types of cartilage (elastic, hyaline, and fibrocartilage) may be involved.
- The most frequently affected sites include the external ears (pinna and external auditory canal), nose, larynx, trachea, proximal bronchial tree, eyes, and large joints.
- Females are affected more than males (3:1), and the median age at diagnosis is in the mid-40s.
- Affected patients present with systemic symptoms (fatigue, fever, and weight loss) and symptoms related to inflammation of the affected cartilaginous structures: in particular, pain in the external ear, nose, and throat; hoarseness; and arthralgia.

- Respiratory tract involvement occurs at some point during the course of the disease in roughly half of affected patients and is the leading cause of death.
- Common findings on CT images include smooth and diffuse thickening and increased attenuation of the trachea and bronchial wall and a variable degree of tracheobronchial wall calcification.
- Occasionally, tracheal or bronchial narrowing occurs.
- Characteristically, only the cartilaginous portion of the tracheal wall is involved; the membranous posterior wall is spared.
- Cylindric bronchiectasis and secondary pulmonary infection may also occur.
- Cardiovascular complications are the second most frequent cause of death and include aortic and mitral valve regurgitation, aortic aneurysm, and myocardial infarction.
- Air trapping and airway collapse (malacia) on expiratory images have been reported in a large proportion of patients with relapsing polychondritis, likely reflecting mucosal edema with cartilaginous inflammation and destruction.

✓ Pearls & ✗ Pitfalls

- ✓ Saddle nose deformity secondary to necrosis and collapse of the cartilaginous nasal septum is another clinical finding associated with relapsing polychondritis.
- ✗ Expiratory CT should be routinely performed in these patients. Examinations in expiration are more sensitive than routine inspiratory CT examinations for demonstrating airway abnormalities in relapsing polychondritis.

Case 35

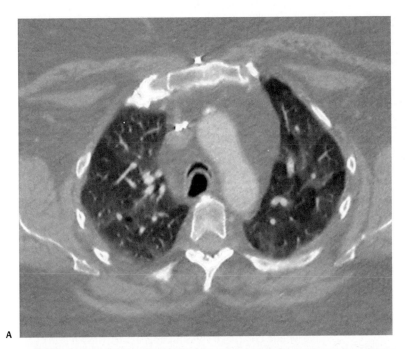

A

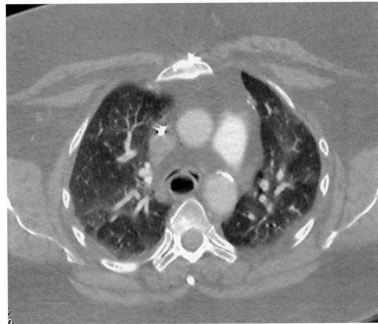

B

▣ Clinical Presentation

A morbidly obese 51-year-old woman, who is a cigarette smoker, with shortness of breath, stridor, and cough.

■ Imaging Findings

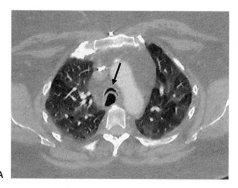
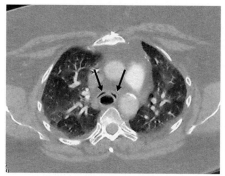

A   B

(A,B) Contrast-enhanced computed tomography of the chest: Expiratory images at two different levels reveal significant collapse of the trachea and airways (*arrows*). Also note the mosaic pattern of attenuation in the lung parenchyma.

■ Differential Diagnosis

- ***Tracheobronchomalacia (TBM):*** Excessive airway collapsibility secondary to weakness of the airway wall is known as TBM.
- *Tracheobronchial stenosis:* A fundamental difference between tracheobronchial stenosis and several different pathologic conditions (amyloidosis, sarcoidosis, relapsing polychondritis) is the fixed nature of the airway narrowing.

■ Essential Facts

- Tracheomalacia (TM) is abnormal weakness of the tracheal wall causing increased collapsibility. TBM is the same process, but with involvement of the upper airways, not only the trachea. The two terms are commonly used interchangeably.
- TM was originally described in children who presented with airway collapse in expiration and clinical manifestations of dyspnea, stridor, and cyanosis.
- In children, TM/TBM may be congenital (primary) or acquired (secondary).
- Congenital TM is commonly associated with prematurity but can be seen in otherwise healthy infants.
- Acquired TM is associated with protracted endotracheal intubation and vascular rings.
- In adults, acquired forms of TBM may result from any condition that damages and weakens the tracheal or bronchial wall: intubation, external trauma, surgery (tracheostomy, lung transplantation), vascular rings and mediastinal tumors (goiter), and inflammation (relapsing polychondritis).
- It has been suggested that cigarette smoking and general chronic inflammation contribute to the development of TBM. More than 20% of adult patients with TBM have chronic bronchitis.

- TBM is not an uncommon condition. It was reported in as many as 20% of patients in a bronchoscopy series.
- Images in expiration show significant anterior bowing of the posterior membranous part of the tracheal wall, bringing the anterior and posterior parts of the tracheal wall closer and creating a crescent appearance (frown sign).

■ Other Imaging Findings

- Dynamic magnetic resonance imaging (MRI) during forced expiration and cough has also been used to evaluate collapsibility of the trachea in TM. The lack of ionizing radiation makes MRI attractive for exploring tracheal morphology during different respiratory maneuvers and for patient follow-up.

✓ Pearls & ✗ Pitfalls

- ✓ A diagnostic criterion for TM commonly used on computed tomography and bronchoscopy is more than 50% tracheal narrowing (cross-sectional area) during expiration.
- ✗ In patients with TM or TBM, images obtained in inspiration may be completely normal or reveal only a lunate configuration and mild degree of tracheomegaly. Because tracheal collapse is most prominent when the intrathoracic pressure is greater than the intraluminal pressure (as it is during expiration, cough, or Valsalva maneuver), images in expiration are usually required to make this diagnosis.

Case 36

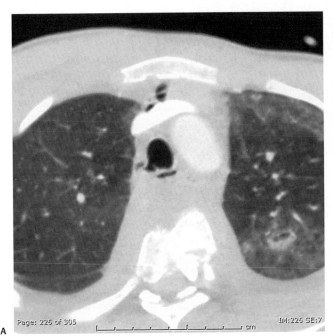

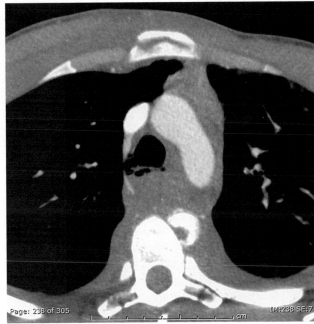

Clinical Presentation

An 18-year-old man after a motor vehicle accident.

■ Imaging Findings

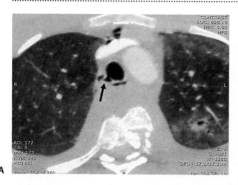 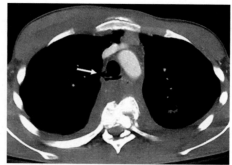

(A,B) Contrast-enhanced computed tomography (CT) of the chest shows a mediastinal hematoma in the posterior mediastinum and paraspinal region, fracture-dislocation of the thoracic spine, and deformity of the right posterior lateral tracheal wall with pneumomediastinum (*arrows*).

■ Differential Diagnosis

- *Tracheal rupture:* Deformity and discontinuity of the tracheal wall with associated pneumomediastinum are consistent with tracheal rupture.
- *Pneumomediastinum without tracheal rupture:* In severe, blunt thoracic trauma, pneumomediastinum may develop without associated tracheobronchial or esophageal rupture.
- *Tracheal diverticulum:* A tracheal diverticulum may be seen as an abnormal collection of air in the right paratracheal region. It should not be associated with pneumomediastinum or subcutaneous emphysema.

■ Essential Facts

- Major tracheobronchial injuries are two times more commonly seen secondary to penetrating trauma than after blunt trauma.
- Tracheobronchial injuries resulting from blunt thoracic trauma are relatively uncommon and found in fewer than 2% of trauma patients.
- Tracheal ruptures comprise one-fourth of all tracheobronchial injuries
- Tracheal rupture is commonly associated with severe blunt trauma and has a high mortality rate (80%).
- Tracheal injury may result from either compression of the sternum against the thoracic spine or a sudden increase of intraluminal pressure against a closed glottis.
- The most common site of tracheal laceration is at the junction of the cartilaginous and membranous portions in the posterolateral wall.
- The typical morphology of tracheal rupture is longitudinal, or vertical. It occurs more commonly in the distal third, close to the carina.

- The most common imaging findings are pneumomediastinum and subcutaneous emphysema (100%), often extending to the neck.
- Pneumothorax can also be present but is relatively uncommon (33%) in isolated tracheal rupture.
- On CT, the tracheal rupture is directly visualized in 70% of cases.
- Esophageal rupture is another uncommon mechanism of pneumomediastinum in patients with blunt trauma.
- In patients with an endotracheal tube, the site of the tracheal laceration may be seen as herniation of the endotracheal balloon, which is present in one-third of affected patients.
- An overly distended endotracheal balloon cuff is another sign of tracheal rupture.

✓ Pearls & ✗ Pitfalls

- ✓ A delay in the diagnosis is the single most important factor adversely influencing the outcome of patients with tracheal rupture. Patients with a delayed diagnosis (> 24 hours) sustain more complications and have a higher mortality rate than do those with early diagnosis and treatment.
- ✗ In trauma patients, the Macklin effect (alveolar rupture and air dissection along bronchovascular sheaths with mediastinal extension) is four times more often the mechanism responsible for pneumomediastinum than tracheobronchial injury.

Case 37

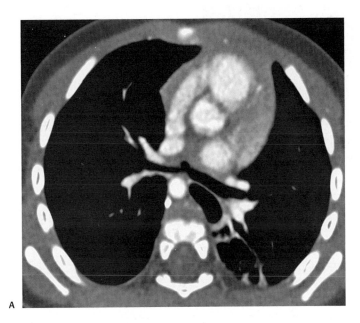

A

Clinical Presentation

A 10-month-old infant with persistent cough and stridor.

Further Work-up

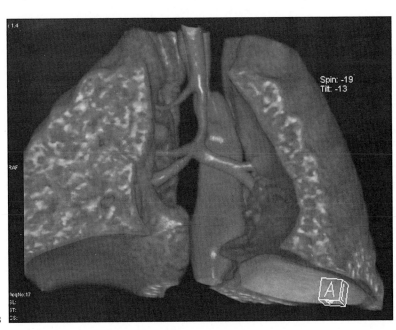

B

■ Imaging Findings

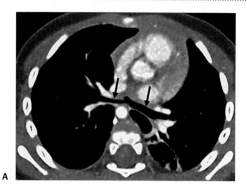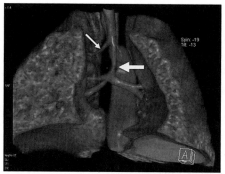

(A,B) Computed tomography (CT) of the chest: axial image at the level of the carina (A) and three-dimensional volume-rendered image (B) show an abnormally long segment of narrowing in the distal tracheal (*thick white arrow*), a horizontal orientation of the bronchi arising from the carina (*black arrows*), and a tracheal bronchus for the right upper lobe (*thin white arrow*).

■ Differential Diagnosis

- ***Long-segment congenital tracheal stenosis:*** Abnormal narrowing of the trachea in an infant with respiratory symptoms, of variable length and commonly associated with an abnormal pattern of tracheobronchial branching, is characteristic of congenital tracheal stenosis.
- *Tracheomalacia:* Respiratory symptoms and tracheal narrowing (dynamic) may also present in children with tracheomalacia.
- *Duplication of the aortic arch:* Vascular rings, like duplication of the aortic arch, may produce tracheal narrowing from extrinsic compression, with respiratory symptoms.

■ Essential Facts

- Congenital tracheal stenosis is commonly secondary to complete cartilaginous tracheal ring, in which the pars membranacea is replaced by cartilaginous tissue, forming a complete "0."
- Approximately 25% of patients with congenital tracheal stenosis also present with aberrant origin of the left pulmonary artery from the right (pulmonary artery sling) and other congenital cardiac defects.
- Patients with pulmonary artery sling commonly present with associated anomalies of the tracheobronchial tree (48–54%).
- The most common are hypoplasia of the distal trachea or right main bronchus, usually associated with complete cartilaginous ring ("napkin ring" cartilage), tracheomalacia, and tracheal bronchus to the right upper lobe (bronchus suis). This constellation of findings is known as the ring-sling complex.

- Other cardiovascular anomalies are also common (> 50%), including persistent left superior vena cava draining into the coronary sinus, atrial septal defect, ventricular septal defect, patent ductus arteriosus, aortic arch anomalies, and tetralogy of Fallot.
- Ninety percent of patients present with respiratory symptoms during the first year of life, the majority at birth or before 6 months of age.
- Chest radiographs may show hyperlucent right lung and deviation of the trachea to the left, with narrowing of the distal tracheal air column.
- Short-segment congenital tracheal stenosis generally has a better prognosis than long-segment stenosis.
- When a pulmonary artery sling is present, a barium esophagogram is often diagnostic, showing an anterior indentation of the esophagus, a finding seen only in this type of vascular ring.

✓ Pearls & ✗ Pitfalls

- ✓ Mortality among patients with aberrant origin of the left pulmonary artery (pulmonary artery sling) and associated tracheobronchial or cardiovascular malformations remains high despite significant improvement with early surgical correction.
- ✗ Vascular rings may present with extrinsic compression of the esophagus and trachea. However, both plain radiographs and the esophagogram are limited in the evaluation of these conditions and in delineating the complex anatomy of such cases. Further evaluation with cross-sectional imaging (CT or magnetic resonance) is required.

Case 38

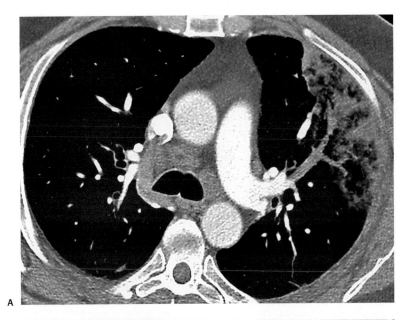

A

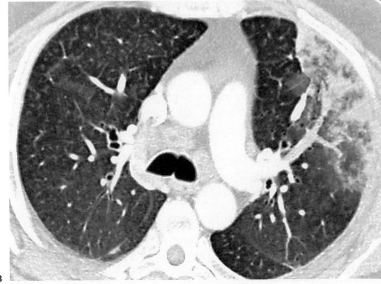

B

■ Clinical Presentation

A 53-year-old man with hemoptysis.

■ Imaging Findings

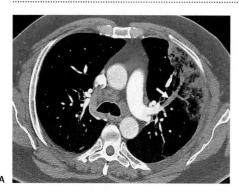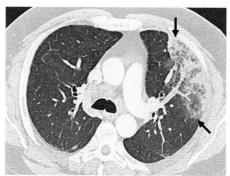

A   B

(A,B) Contrast-enhanced computed tomography (CT): axial images in mediastinal (A) and lung (B) windows demonstrate a pleura-based triangular opacity extending from the right hilum (*black arrows*), as well as the absence of contrast opacification in a segmental branch of the left upper lobe pulmonary artery (*white arrow*).

■ Differential Diagnosis

• ***Pulmonary infarct secondary to acute pulmonary embolism (PE):*** A triangular pleura-based parenchymal opacity, usually with air-space consolidation and a filling defect of the pulmonary artery supplying that portion of the lung, is characteristic of a lung infarct.
• *PE and independent pulmonary parenchymal disease:* A pulmonary artery embolism can be seen involving a lung previously affected with lung cancer or pneumonia.
• *Atelectasis:* A parenchymal opacity resulting from atelectasis may be triangular in shape and exhibit an air bronchogram.

■ Essential Facts

• Nonspecific parenchymal abnormalities are common (> 85%) in patients with PE.
• Atelectasis and focal areas of parenchymal opacity are the most common findings.
• In a small number of patients with PE, the parenchymal changes are more severe, with hemorrhage and occasionally some degree of tissue necrosis.
• The area of parenchymal opacity is typically fairly well demarcated and triangular or wedge-shaped. It extends to the periphery, abutting the pleura.
• The predominant histologic finding is parenchymal hemorrhage.
• On CT, these areas appear as ground-glass density, parenchymal consolidation, or a mixture of both.
• Associated pleural effusion is common.

• In the chronic stage, the area of hemorrhage is replaced by scar, with the development of a nodular or elongated scar, linear atelectatic band, and some degree of pleural thickening.
• The triangular parenchymal opacity resulting from a pulmonary infarct, which resembles a pleura-based truncated cone on images, is known as Hampton's hump.
• In the subacute stage, the liberation of enzymes from neutrophils in the hemorrhagic area may produce cavity formation as the result of liquefaction of the hemorrhagic and necrotic tissue.
• On chest CT, the appearance of central lucencies within a peripheral consolidation favors a pulmonary infarction.

✓ Pearls & ✗ Pitfalls

✓ Besides embolism, pulmonary infarction may also result from lung cancer, metastasis, surgery, and in general any condition that impairs the normal flow through either the pulmonary arteries or pulmonary veins.
✗ The parenchymal opacity seen on chest radiographs resulting from pulmonary infarction and hemorrhage secondary to PE is a nonspecific finding. A similar appearance may be seen in pneumonia, atelectasis, and even a neoplastic process.

Case 39

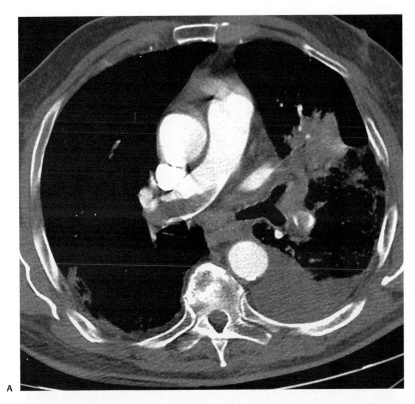

A

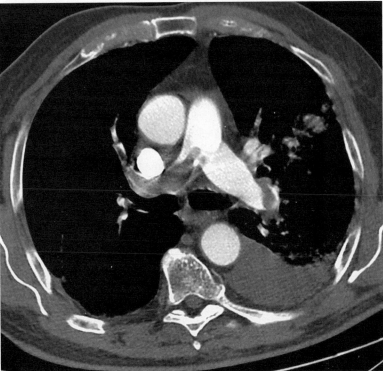

B

■ Clinical Presentation

Routine follow-up computed tomography of the chest in a patient with known lung cancer and no new or acute respiratory symptoms.

■ Imaging Findings

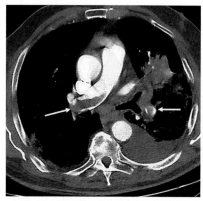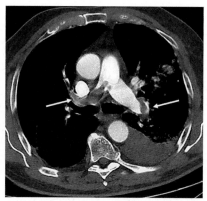

A   B

(A,B) Contrast-enhanced computed tomography (CT) of the chest: Axial images at the level of the pulmonary hila demonstrate large filling defects in the right and left pulmonary arteries (*arrows*). An irregular soft-tissue-density mass is seen in relation to the left hilum, as well as a moderately sized ipsilateral pleural effusion.

■ Differential Diagnosis

- ***Pulmonary embolism (PE):*** Large filling defects in the pulmonary arteries, like those in this patient, are consistent with PE.
- *Metastatic embolism:* Distant malignancies can occasionally produce nonthrombotic tumoral embolism to the pulmonary vasculature.

■ Essential Facts

- Malignancy and chemotherapy are independent risk factors associated with an increased risk for venous thrombosis and PE.
- Unsuspected PE is detected in 1.5% of routine contrast-enhanced CT scans of the chest.
- The rate of incidental PE is even higher in oncology patients, of whom 4% will have PE on routine CT examination.
- Unsuspected iliofemoral deep venous thrombosis is reported in almost 7% of oncology patients.
- The prevalence of PE in patients with a history of malignancy has been reported to be highest in those with gynecologic malignancies (15%), followed by those with melanoma (10%).

- Other tumors known to be associated with an increased incidence of venous thromboembolism are cancers of the breast, colon, pancreas, and lung.
- Similarly, a primary episode of deep venous thrombosis or PE is associated with an increased risk for a subsequent diagnosis of cancer (odds ratio, 2.3 after a first episode and 4.3 after recurrent episodes).
- In 50% of cancer patients with PE, multiple lobes are involved.
- Pitfalls in the diagnosis of PE in oncology patients result from important confounding factors, such as parenchymal masses, atelectasis, lymphadenopathy, and pleural effusion.

✓ Pearls & ✗ Pitfalls

- ✓ Patients with cancer and associated venous thromboembolism have a worse prognosis and a lower survival rate than those with cancer and no thrombosis.
- ✗ Up to 75% of PEs that are evident on CT examinations in oncology patients are not diagnosed during the initial interpretation of the routine examination. Interestingly, 75% of patients with a diagnosis of unsuspected PE do not have clinical symptoms or signs of venous thromboembolism.

Case 40

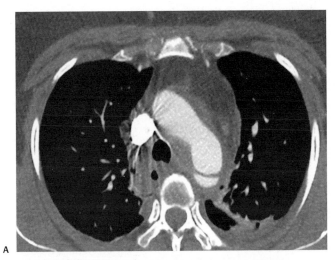
A

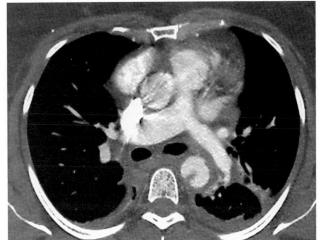
B

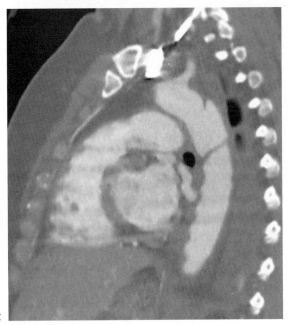
C

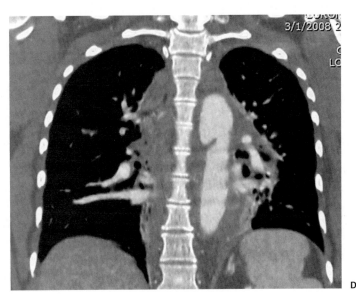
D

■ Clinical Presentation

....

A 43-year-old man with chest pain after a motor vehicle accident.

■ Imaging Findings

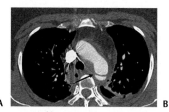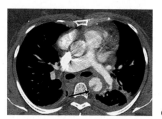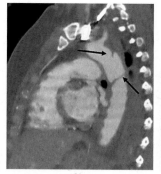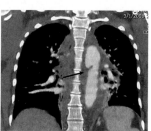

A   B   C   D

(A–D) Contrast-enhanced thoracic computed tomography (CT): Axial images (A,B) and sagittal and coronal re-formations (C,D) demonstrate an abnormal appearance of the distal aortic arch and proximal descending aorta, an intimal flap, and abnormal change in the aortic caliber (*arrows*). Abnormal density of the mediastinum, consistent with mediastinal hematoma, is noted.

■ Differential Diagnosis

- **Traumatic aortic injury (TAI):** In approximately 90% of cases, TAI occurs in the region of the aortic isthmus, just distal to the origin of the left subclavian artery. The combination of a mediastinal hematoma in contact with the aorta and an irregularity of the aortic wall resulting from a pseudoaneurysm or an intimal flap confirms the diagnosis.
- *Non-aortic bleeding and hematoma:* In ~80% of trauma patients with mediastinal hematomas, the bleeding is non-aortic in nature. When the hematoma is confined to the anterior mediastinum, a sternal fracture is usually responsible; when the hematoma is in the posterior mediastinum, a vertebral fracture is usually the source of bleeding.
- *Atherosclerotic saccular aneurysm of the aorta:* In such cases, the aortic contour is abnormal because of the aneurysm, but typically no periaortic hematoma is present, except if there is leaking. The finding of calcium at the level of the aneurysm favors a chronic atherosclerotic lesion.

■ Essential Facts

- Traumatic aortic rupture is the cause of death in 15% of persons who die in motor vehicle accidents.
- A wide mediastinum in a trauma victim should raise the concern for a mediastinal hematoma. In both motor vehicle accident victims and persons with a penetrating thoracic injury, the possibility of a vascular injury should always be the first consideration.
- Between 70% and 85% of TAIs are fatal at the scene of trauma.
- Of the remaining short-term survivors, half die within the first 24 hours.

- A rapid deceleration injury or blunt chest trauma should arouse suspicion of aortic injury.
- The aortic isthmus, which is the portion of the descending thoracic aorta between the origin of the left subclavian artery and the site of attachment of the ligamentum arteriosum, is where most TAIs occur. Some consider tethering of the aorta by the ligamentum arteriosum to be a contributing factor.
- Mediastinal hemorrhage is highly sensitive but less specific for the diagnosis of TAI.
- The combination of a mediastinal hematoma in contact with the aortic wall and a contour deformity of the aorta (e.g., pseudoaneurysm, intimal tear, intraluminal thrombus, or pseudo-coarctation) is the most reliable sign to make this diagnosis.

■ Other Imaging Findings

- Catheter aortography may be needed if the results of helical CT of the aorta are indeterminate or inadequate to exclude injury, or to confirm and define the extent of injury before surgery or endovascular repair.

✓ Pearls & ✗ Pitfalls

- ✓ Contrast-enhanced CT has 100% sensitivity and 100% negative predictive value for the detection of TAI.
- ✗ Diagnostic pitfalls may result from residual thymic tissue or atelectasis mimicking a mediastinal hematoma, from streak or pulsation artifacts, or from a patent ductus arteriosus that may mimic an abnormal aortic wall.

Case 41

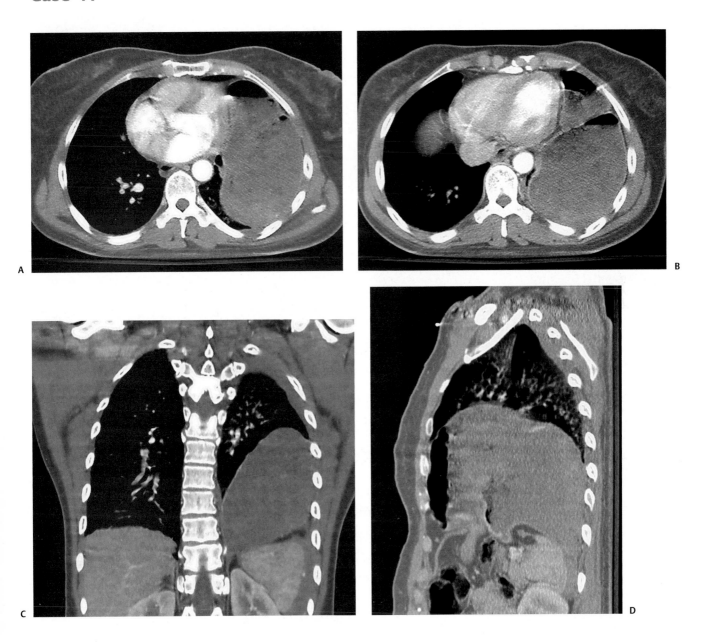

A

B

C

D

Clinical Presentation

A 52-year-old woman with abnormal chest radiographic findings after a motor vehicle accident.

Imaging Findings

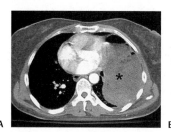 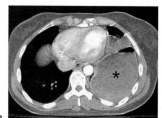 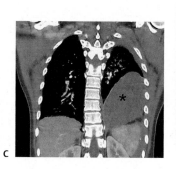 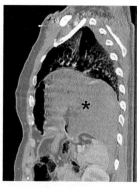

A   B   C   D

(A–D) Contrast-enhanced computed tomography (CT) of the chest: Axial (A,B), sagittal (C), and coronal (D) images demonstrate a distended stomach and a large air-fluid level in the left hemithorax in intimate relation with the left posterior ribs (*asterisks*). Ill-defined ground-glass parenchymal opacities are also noted diffusely affecting the left lung.

Differential Diagnosis

- *Left diaphragmatic rupture:* On CT, in a trauma patient who is supine, an intra-abdominal viscus lying immediately anterior to the posterior ribs is consistent with a ruptured diaphragm.
- *Congenital diaphragmatic hernia:* Congenital left-sided diaphragmatic hernias typically present in neonates and are associated with severe respiratory distress. Smaller diaphragmatic defects can be seen in adults and may be an incidental finding with no clinical manifestations.
- *Diaphragmatic eventration:* Eventration of the diaphragm is a congenital partial or complete failure in the development of the diaphragm. It usually affects the left side. A thin, membranous diaphragm is the result, usually with significant elevation and decreased respiratory motion.

Essential Facts

- Diaphragmatic injuries occur in fewer than 10% of patients with severe thoracoabdominal injury and are commonly associated (> 50%) with other significant traumatic injuries (e.g., pelvic fracture, splenic laceration, and traumatic aortic injury).
- Typically, affected patients are young adult men (average age, 38 years).
- The morbidity and mortality associated with traumatic diaphragmatic rupture are significant (> 30%) and result mainly from the other, concomitant traumatic lesions.
- Gastrointestinal strangulation complicating unrecognized diaphragmatic rupture and visceral herniation may have a high mortality rate (60%).
- The difference in pressure between the peritoneal cavity and the pleural cavity favors intrathoracic herniation of the abdominal contents, which over time tends to enlarge the diaphragmatic defect.

- With the "dependent viscera" sign, the cranial aspect of an abdominal viscus (stomach or colon on the left, liver on the right) is seen lying immediately on top of the posterior ribs because of the lack of diaphragmatic support.
- Diaphragmatic injuries from blunt trauma are usually large, and the mechanism of rupture is related to the large sudden increase in intra-abdominal pressure.
- CT has 84% sensitivity and 77% specificity in the detection and diagnosis of diaphragmatic injury.

Other Imaging Findings

- Other imaging findings are those associated with diaphragmatic rupture and include apparent elevation of the diaphragm, visualization of intra-abdominal contents in the thorax, waistlike constriction of the herniated viscus (collar sign), direct visualization of the diaphragmatic defect, and a thickened diaphragmatic crus.

✓ Pearls & ✗ Pitfalls

- ✓ Diaphragmatic injuries from blunt trauma are three times more common on the left than on the right, likely because of a protective effect of the liver on the right side. Diaphragmatic injuries from penetrating trauma are more evenly distributed between the two sides.
- ✗ Between 60% and 75% of patients with traumatic diaphragmatic rupture present with the intrathoracic herniation of intra-abdominal organs. In those without herniation, recognition of the injury on initial imaging examinations may be more difficult.

Case 42

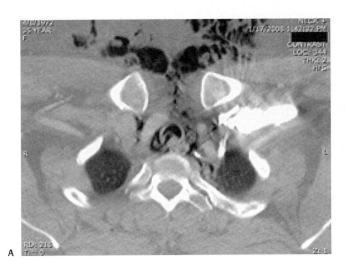 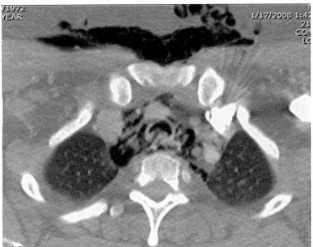

A   B

■ Clinical Presentation

A 35-year-old morbidly obese woman with chest pain after a motor vehicle accident.

■ Imaging Findings

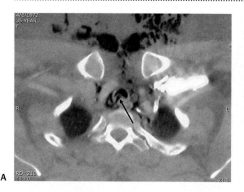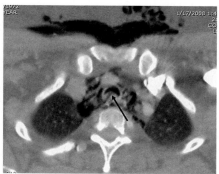

(A,B) Contrast-enhanced computed tomography (CT) of the chest shows significant subcutaneous and mediastinal emphysema, as well as irregularity and a thin, linear, air-density band in relation to the posterior tracheal wall (*arrows*).

■ Differential Diagnosis

- **Tracheal rupture:** Deformity and discontinuity of the tracheal wall associated with pneumomediastinum are consistent with tracheal rupture.
- *Pneumomediastinum without tracheal rupture:* In severe blunt thoracic trauma, pneumomediastinum may develop without associated tracheobronchial or esophageal rupture.
- *Tracheal diverticulum:* A tracheal diverticulum may be seen as an abnormal collection of air in the right paratracheal region, but it should not be associated with pneumomediastinum or subcutaneous emphysema.

■ Essential Facts

- Tracheal ruptures comprise one-fourth of all tracheobronchial injuries.
- Tracheal rupture is commonly associated with severe blunt trauma and has a high mortality rate (80%).
- Tracheal injury may result from either compression of the sternum against the thoracic spine or a sudden increase of intraluminal pressure against a closed glottis.
- The most common site of tracheal laceration is at the junction of the cartilaginous and membranous portions in the posterolateral wall.
- The typical morphology of tracheal rupture is longitudinal, or vertical. It occurs more commonly in the distal third, close to the carina.
- The most common imaging findings are pneumomediastinum and subcutaneous emphysema (100%), often extending to the neck.

- Pneumothorax can also be present but is relatively uncommon (33%) in isolated tracheal rupture.
- On CT, tracheal rupture is directly visualized in only 70% of cases.
- Esophageal rupture is another uncommon mechanism of pneumomediastinum in patients with blunt trauma.
- In patients with an endotracheal tube, the site of the tracheal laceration may be seen as herniation of the endotracheal balloon, a finding present in one-third of affected patients.
- An overly distended endotracheal balloon cuff is another sign of tracheal rupture.

✓ Pearls & ✗ Pitfalls

- ✓ A delay in the diagnosis is the single most important factor adversely influencing the outcome of patients with tracheal rupture. Patients with a delayed diagnosis (> 24 hours) sustain more complications and have a higher mortality rate than those with early diagnosis and treatment.
- ✗ In trauma patients, the Macklin effect (alveolar rupture and air dissection along bronchovascular sheaths with mediastinal extension) is four times more often the mechanism responsible for pneumomediastinum than tracheobronchial injury.

Case 43

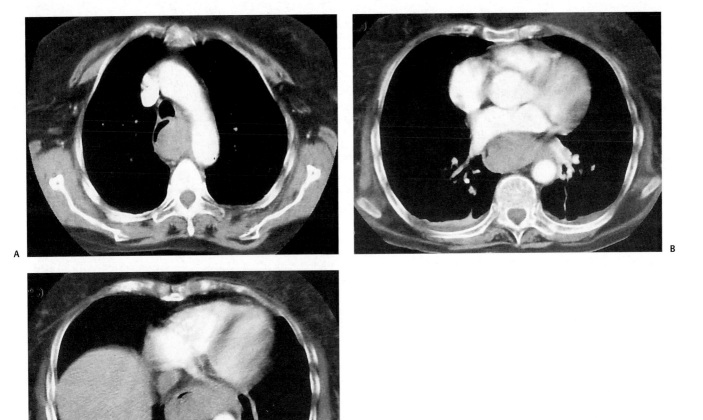

A

B

C

■ Clinical Presentation

A 53-year-old woman with a past medical history of anticoagulation therapy for pulmonary embolism and deep vein thrombosis, now presenting with acute chest pain.

■ Imaging Findings

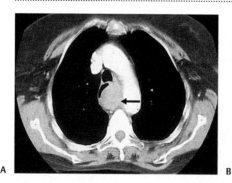 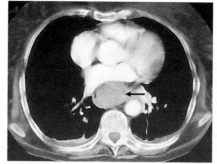 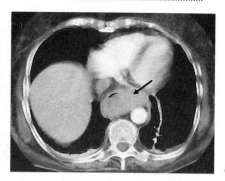

(A–C) Contrast-enhanced computed tomography (CT) of the chest: axial images demonstrate a large, well-defined hyperdensity throughout the entire length of the esophageal wall, eccentrically located and displacing the lumen anteriorly and to the right (*arrows*).

■ Differential Diagnosis

- ***Intramural hematoma of the esophagus (IHE):*** Acute IHE may present as a hyperdense collection located either concentrically or eccentrically in the esophageal wall.
- *Esophageal tumor:* Abnormal wall thickening or soft-tissue density in relation to the esophageal wall can represent an esophageal tumor.
- *Mediastinal hematoma:* Mediastinal hematoma (e.g., paraspinal hemorrhagic collection from vertebral fracture or aortic injury) may present as a hyperdense collection adjacent to the esophagus.

■ Essential Facts

- IHE consists of a submucosal collection of blood within the layers of the esophageal wall.
- The distal esophagus is more commonly affected, but involvement of the entire esophagus is also possible.
- IHE can result from different mechanisms; abnormal hemostasis (hemophilia, thrombocytopenia, anticoagulation therapy), emetogenesis (vomiting, retching), and trauma are the most common.
- The most common cause of IHE is abnormal hemostasis, which is responsible in approximately one-third of cases.
- In those cases associated with vomiting, intrathoracic hyperpressure is considered to be responsible for a submucosal tear, which produces bleeding and intramural dissection of the esophageal wall.
- Eighteen percent of cases are considered to develop from a submucosal tear.

- Iatrogenic cases associated with diagnostic or therapeutic endoscopic procedures are also well documented.
- Adult patients of all ages have been reported, with an average age of about 58 years.
- Chest pain, odynophagia, and dysphagia are the typical clinical problems.
- On CT, a nonenhancing eccentric or concentric mass or thickening in the esophageal wall is characteristic.
- The measured blood density and attenuation of an IHE vary according to its age, from hyperdense in the acute stage to hypodense in the subacute stage.
- The posterior esophageal wall is the most commonly involved.
- When there is communication between the intramural dissection and the esophageal lumen, an oral contrast esophagogram reveals a striplike accumulation of contrast ("double-barrel" sign), which is considered diagnostic of this condition.

✓ Pearls & ✗ Pitfalls

- ✓ Hematemesis is an uncommon initial symptom, in contrast to Mallory-Weiss tear, in which there is a superficial mucosal tear. Ultimately, hematemesis develops in roughly half of affected patients when the expanding hematoma finally penetrates through the submucosa into the esophageal lumen.
- ✗ When an IHE is confined to the esophageal wall, without an associated mucosal tear, a contrast esophagogram may be limited in demonstrating the size, nature, and extent of the esophageal wall abnormality.

Case 44

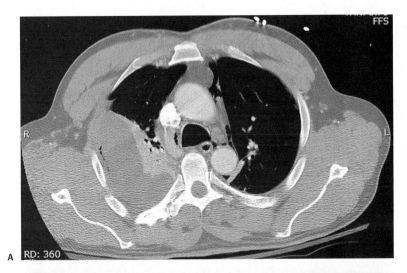

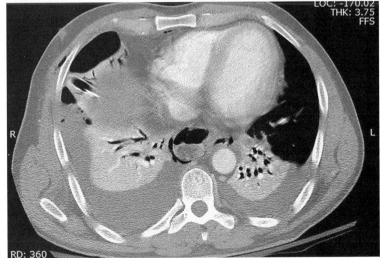

Clinical Presentation

A 40-year-old man with acute chest pain after an alcohol binge.

■ Imaging Findings

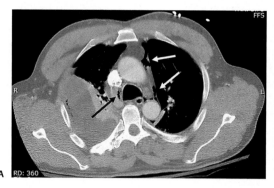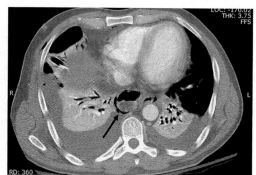

(A,B) Contrast-enhanced computed tomography (CT) of the chest demonstrates pneumomediastinum, with air in the middle mediastinum (*arrows*, A) and surrounding the distal esophagus at the level of the esophagogastric junction (*arrow*, B). Bilateral pleural effusions and bilateral basilar parenchymal opacities are also appreciated.

■ Differential Diagnosis

- **Boerhaave syndrome:** The development of pneumomediastinum, effusion, and hydropneumothorax after an episode of forceful vomiting suggests esophageal rupture.
- *Tracheobronchial injury:* Pneumomediastinum is always concerning for the presence of tracheobronchial injury, which in trauma patients can be associated with pleural air and fluid.
- *Acute mediastinitis:* Mediastinal air and fluid can be seen in infective mediastinitis resulting from a variety of conditions, such as posterior mediastinal extension of a retropharyngeal abscess, postsurgical complications, and esophageal and airway injuries, among others.

■ Essential Facts

- Boerhaave syndrome refers to the "spontaneous" perforation of the esophagus during instrumentation or external trauma. It is typically associated with forceful vomiting and/or retching.
- The mechanism responsible for the esophageal rupture is likely related to the sudden increase of intraluminal pressure.
- Pain is the presenting symptom in the majority of patients (85%), followed by vomiting (71%).
- The diagnosis should be suspected in the presence of the Mackler triad: vomiting, strong and sudden chest pain, and subcutaneous emphysema.

- Other presenting symptoms include shock, fever, jaundice, dyspnea, and back pain.
- The most common site of perforation is on the left side of the distal esophagus.
- Imaging manifestations include pneumomediastinum with periesophageal air, pleural effusion (bilaterally or on the left side), pneumothorax, and pneumopericardium.
- A delayed diagnosis is associated with a high rate of mortality from polymicrobial mediastinitis and sepsis.
- Contrast esophagography or CT after the oral administration of contrast demonstrates extravasation of the contrast medium at a supradiaphragmatic or subdiaphragmatic level.

✓ Pearls & ✗ Pitfalls

- ✓ "Spontaneous" rupture of the esophagus has also been described in other situations and conditions in which the intraluminal pressure increases suddenly, such as weightlifting, coughing, hiccups, childbirth, seizures, and straining.
- ✗ Boerhaave syndrome is commonly misdiagnosed as myocardial infarction, aortic dissection, pulmonary embolism, pancreatitis, or perforated peptic ulcer.

Case 45

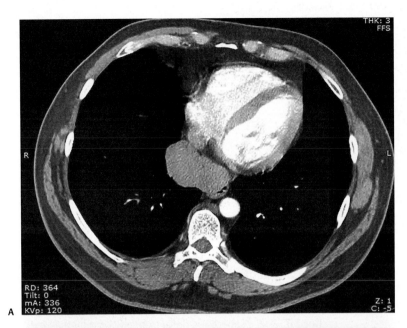

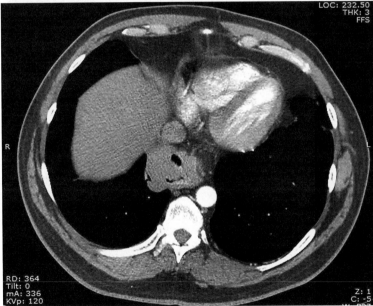

◼ Clinical Presentation

A 52-year-old man with dysphagia.

Imaging Findings

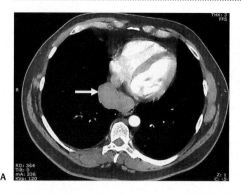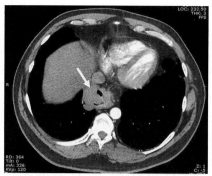

(A,B) Contrast-enhanced thoracic computed tomography (CT) reveals a well-defined soft-tissue-density mediastinal mass eccentrically located in the distal esophagus (*arrows*). There is a clear interface with adjacent structures with no obvious infiltrative changes.

Differential Diagnosis

- ***Esophageal leiomyoma:*** A well-defined soft-tissue-density mass in the distal esophagus may represent an esophageal leiomyoma.
- *Esophageal fibroma/schwannoma:* Other benign esophageal tumors (e.g., fibromas and schwannomas) have identical imaging appearances, presenting as noninfiltrative soft-tissue mass.
- *Esophageal carcinoma:* An abnormal mass arising from the esophageal wall should raise concern for the possibility of an esophageal carcinoma.

Essential Facts

- Leiomyoma is the most common benign esophageal tumor, accounting for more than 60% of benign neoplasms arising from the esophagus.
- Leiomyomas are well-encapsulated tumors composed of a mixture of benign smooth muscle and fibrous tissue.
- They may be multiple in 5% of patients.
- The most common location of esophageal leiomyomas is in the distal esophagus (> 60%), followed by the middle third (30%). Involvement of the upper esophagus is uncommon (10%).
- These are slowly growing submucosal lesions that are commonly asymptomatic.
- When symptoms develop, the most common are epigastric discomfort and dysphagia.
- Symptomatic patients are on average about 45 years old, and men are more commonly affected than women (2:1).

- Ulceration and bleeding are less common with esophageal than with gastric leiomyomas.
- On CT, they appear as round or lobulated soft-tissue masses that are homogeneous in density, with a well-defined interface separating them from adjacent mediastinal structures.
- Large esophageal leiomyomas appear on chest radiographs as mediastinal masses, typically in the retrocardiac region.
- These tumors are generally enucleated without any need for esophageal resection (97%).

Other Imaging Findings

- Magnetic resonance imaging allows a better determination of the submucosal location of these tumors so that they can be differentiated from mucosal lesions like carcinomas.

✓ Pearls & ✗ Pitfalls

- ✓ Esophageal leiomyomatosis may be associated with Alport syndrome, an X-linked genetic condition in which a genetic mutation prevents the proper biosynthesis of type IV collagen. Diffuse leiomyomatosis of the esophagus, female genitalia, or both may be present in this condition. Other findings include nephritis, hematuria, sensorineural hearing loss, and cataracts.
- ✗ CT cannot differentiate between leiomyomas and noninvasive esophageal carcinomas. All soft-tissue-density masses detected on CT should be further evaluated with upper gastrointestinal endoscopy.

Case 46

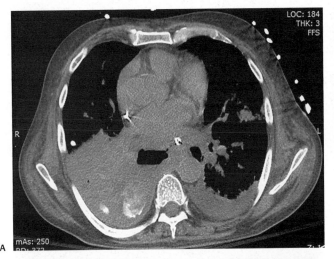

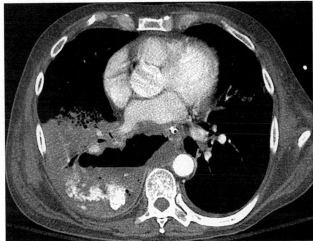

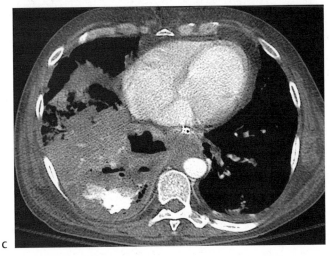

■ Clinical Presentation

....

A 64-year-old man with cough, fever, and weight loss.

■ Imaging Findings

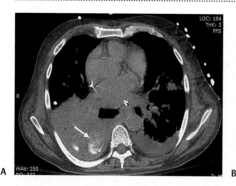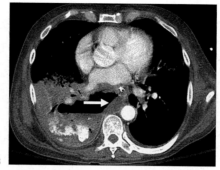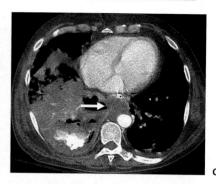

(A–C) Computed tomography (CT) of the chest after administration of oral contrast (A) shows a large parenchymal opacity with central cavitation and an air-fluid level in the right lower lobe with an accumulation of oral contrast (*arrow*, A). An abnormal soft-tissue mass is noted between the esophagus, posterior aspect of the left atrium, and descending thoracic aorta, better appreciated on the contrast-enhanced images (*arrows*, B,C).

■ Differential Diagnosis

- ***Esophagopulmonary fistula:*** An abnormal accumulation of orally administered contrast in the lung parenchyma may result from the presence of a fistulous tract between the esophagus and the tracheobronchial tree.
- *Aspiration:* The abnormal aspiration of gastric contents may also result in an accumulation of oral contrast in the lung parenchyma.
- *Esophageal perforation and mediastinal abscess:* In the presence of mediastinal perforation, oral contrast can be seen abnormally accumulated in the mediastinum and, depending on the level of the perforation, extending into the pleural space and even the peritoneal cavity.

■ Essential Facts

- The majority of esophageal fistulas seen in adult patients result from acquired diseases, such as intrathoracic malignancies (> 60%)—in particular, esophageal cancer (77%), followed by lung cancer (16%).
- Causes of fistulas between the esophagus and respiratory tract other than malignancy are trauma, medical instrumentation (endoscopy and stent placement), chemical injury, prolonged intubation, and infection (tuberculosis).
- A fistulous tract may develop between the esophagus and the trachea, lungs, and bronchi.
- Advanced esophageal carcinomas (T4) result in fistulas between the esophagus and respiratory tract in up to 15% of cases.

- The incidence of fistula formation also increases with radiation therapy.
- The initial clinical presentation is recurrent pneumonia with a variable degree of parenchymal consolidation secondary to aspiration and sepsis.
- CT after the oral administration of contrast reveals an abnormal accumulation of contrast in the airways or lung parenchyma.
- If necrotizing pneumonia develops, oral contrast may accumulate within the necrotizing cavity.
- Esophagopleural fistula may also develop secondary to esophageal cancer (T4).

✓ Pearls & ✗ Pitfalls

- ✓ The prognosis of patients with esophageal cancer and a fistula between the esophagus and respiratory tract is extremely poor, with an approximately 1-month survival. Palliative measures improve the quality of life of affected patients without significantly modifying outcome.
- ✗ Cross-sectional imaging is limited for defining the exact morphology of the fistula. Fluoroscopic esophagography is usually required to confirm the diagnosis and define the exact location and extent of the fistulous tract.

Case 47

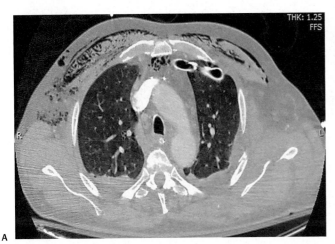

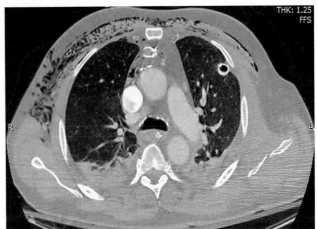

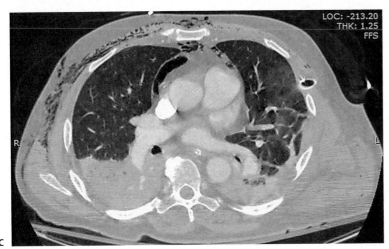

■ Clinical Presentation

Adult patient with severe chest pain and worsening subcutaneous emphysema after placement of chest tube for left-sided pneumothorax.

■ Imaging Findings

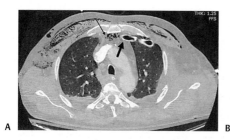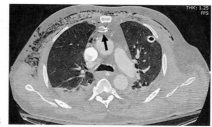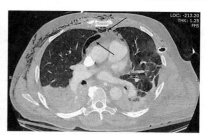

A   B   C

(A–C) Computed tomography (CT) of the chest: Axial images at three different levels demonstrate a left-sided thoracostomy tube with its tip within the fat of the anterior mediastinum (*thick black arrows*), as well as a significant degree of pneumomediastinum and subcutaneous emphysema (*thin black arrows*). Bilateral parenchymal opacities are also noted.

■ Differential Diagnosis

- ***Malposition of a thoracostomy tube:*** Thoracostomy tubes placed for the evacuation of a pneumothorax or pleural fluid should be within the pleural space. When the tube tip is within the mediastinum, the mediastinal pleura has been violated, resulting in various complications.
- *Mediastinal chest tube:* After cardiac surgery, thoracostomy tubes are placed in the mediastinum to prevent the accumulation of blood and rapidly detect active bleeding. These tubes are more commonly placed in a vertical orientation in the retrosternal region, with the exit point beneath the sternum, inferiorly.
- *Normally positioned thoracostomy tube:* The ideal position of a thoracostomy tube for the drainage of a pneumothorax is in the upper anterior pleural space.

■ Essential Facts

- Closed thoracostomy tubes are very commonly placed in either an elective or an emergent procedure to evacuate air and fluid in the pleural cavity.
- After placement, the tube position should be confirmed with conventional chest radiography.
- When adhesions or loculated pleural effusions are present, CT guidance or ultrasound assistance may be needed for proper tube placement.
- Thoracostomy tubes are usually recommended when pneumothorax is associated with lung collapse of more than 25%.
- Other common indications for the placement of thoracostomy tubes are to drain empyema, large recurrent pleural effusions, hemothorax, and malignant effusions.

- Tubes are commonly placed in an intercostal space between the 4th and 9th ribs, in the anterior chest wall, or in the mid-clavicular or anterior axillary line.
- For the drainage of a pneumothorax, an anterior location of the tube is preferred, whereas for the drainage of fluid, a posterior position is preferred.
- Emergency tube placement results in a high incidence of complications (25%), with improper position the most common.
- Malposition of tubes in extrathoracic (in the soft tissues of the chest wall or intra-abdominally), intramediastinal, intrafissural, or intraparenchymal locations or in the thoracic inlet with subclavian vessel injury may occur.
- Chest tube malposition is associated with increased morbidity and mortality.
- Hepatic laceration and splenic laceration are the two most common visceral injuries resulting from chest tube malposition.

✓ Pearls & ✗ Pitfalls

- ✓ Emergency placement of a thoracostomy tube is associated with a relatively high incidence of tube malposition and complications, the diagnosis of which is more limited with conventional radiography than with CT.
- ✗ The tube position relative to air or fluid can be misleading in a single anteroposterior view and can be better defined in a lateral projection.

Case 48

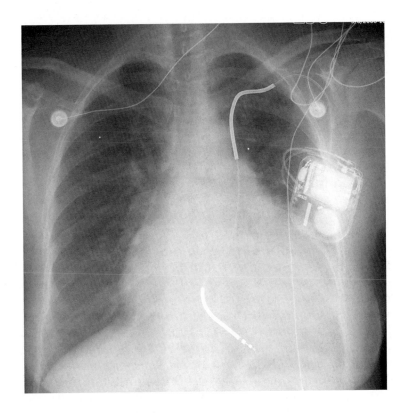

■ Clinical Presentation

Chest radiograph from an adult patient after a cardiac intervention.

■ Imaging Findings

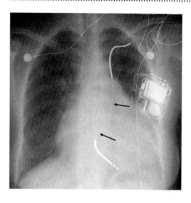

Single anteroposterior (AP) radiograph of the chest shows the lead of the pacing device coursing from a left subclavian approach to the left of midline and terminating in the usual position for the right ventricle (*arrows*). A significantly enlarged cardiac silhouette with a left ventricular configuration is also appreciated.

■ Differential Diagnosis

- ***Persistent left superior vena cava (PLSVC):*** PLSVC is typically found incidentally on a chest radiograph obtained after a placement of a left-sided central venous line or during contrast-enhanced computed tomography. Occasionally, a conventional chest radiograph may show mild mediastinal widening with a soft-tissue density to the left of the aortic knob. On cross-sectional images, the PLSVC is seen as a vascular structure connecting the confluence of the left subclavian vein and internal jugular vein with the coronary sinus.
- *Partial anomalous pulmonary venous return (PAPVR):* A large venous structure can also be seen to the left of the aortic arch in patients with a PAPVR of the left upper lobe, but it will typically connect to the brachiocephalic vein, not to the coronary sinus, and the venous drainage from the lung parenchyma will be different from that of a PLSVC.
- *Malposition of an automatic implantable cardioverter defibrillator (AICD) lead:* Leads from pacemakers and implantable defibrillators may be malpositioned in the pleural space or mediastinum, or in an unexpected vessel.

■ Essential Facts

- AICDs are devices implanted in the chest wall to monitor and, if required, correct episodes of cardiac arrhythmia (e.g., ventricular tachycardia with a cardiac rate > 175 beats per minute), or to restore sinus rhythm in cases of ventricular fibrillation.
- Cardioversion is the conversion of one rhythm to another. It may be used to correct ventricular fibrillation.
- An AICD is similar in many aspects to a pacemaker. Pacemakers are typically used to control bradyarrhythmias, whereas AICDs are used more for the treatment of tachyarrhythmias, although they are also effective for anti-bradycardia pacing.
- Both pacemakers and AICDs consist of three parts: (1) a generator with lithium batteries and a small computer processor; (2) leads or wires made of platinum with an

insulating coat (silicone or polyurethane), which carry the electric impulses and relay information back from the heart to the generator; and (3) electrodes, which are tiny devices at the tip of the lead that deliver the electric impulse to the myocardium.
- The generator is placed in a prepectoral position (above the pectoralis muscle), and the leads are placed transvenously, usually via a subclavian vein.
- Operative mortality with a transvenous (nonthoracotomy) AICD is less than 1%, and the infection rate is ~2%.
- Other complications of pacing devices include bacterial endocarditis, myocardial perforation, venous thrombosis and superior vena cava syndrome, lead malposition or migration, lead fracture, pacemaker box erosion, pneumothorax, and pericardial effusion.
- Depending on the patient's need, one, two, or three leads are typically placed in (1) a single cardiac chamber (single-chamber AICD); (2) two different cardiac chambers, such as the right atrium and right ventricle; or (3) both ventricles or three chambers (right atrium, right ventricle, and left ventricle).

✓ Pearls & ✗ Pitfalls

- ✓ Whether magnetic resonance imaging (MRI) should be considered absolutely contraindicated in patients with an AICD remains controversial. Pacemaker and AICD labeling currently cautions physicians and patients against the use of MRI. Although several studies report that arrhythmia induction from MRI is a rare event, the potential for such events exists, and the consequences can be catastrophic. Lithotripsy is also contraindicated if the pulse generator is the field.
- ✗ A single AP view of the chest is limited for evaluating the exact position of the lead and distal electrode of a pacing device, which can be better evaluated with both an AP and a posteroanterior or lateral projection.

Case 49

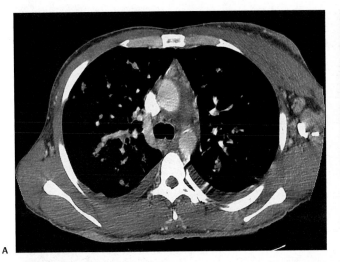
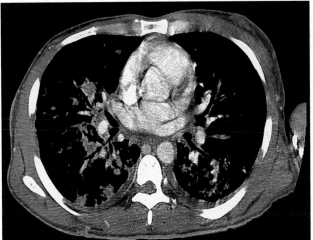

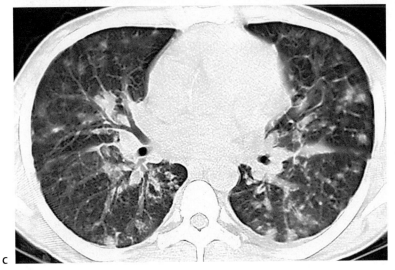

■ Clinical Presentation

A human immunodeficiency virus–positive young adult man with progressive shortness of breath and cough.

■ Imaging Findings

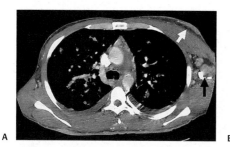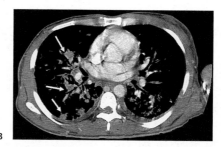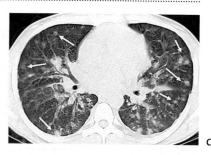

(A–C) Contrast-enhanced computed tomography of the chest: Mediastinal window images (A,B) demonstrate enlarged lymph nodes in the mediastinum and left axilla, as well as skin thickening and nodularity of the anterior chest wall (*arrows*, A). Abnormal peribronchovascular thickening and enlarged hilar lymph nodes, as well as hazy nodules scattered throughout the lung parenchyma, are better appreciated in the lung window image (*arrows*, C).

■ Differential Diagnosis

- **Kaposi sarcoma (KS):** Bilateral pulmonary nodules in a peribronchovascular distribution associated with enhancing lymphadenopathy and skin thickening in a human immunodeficiency virus (HIV)–positive patient are suggestive of lung involvement from KS.
- *Lymphoma:* Multicentric non-Hodgkin lymphoma may also manifest as enlarged lymph nodes, multiple pulmonary nodules, and peribronchovascular opacities with a variable degree of pleural effusion.
- *Opportunistic infection:* Tuberculosis and atypical mycobacterial and other opportunistic infections (e.g., *Pneumocystis jiroveci, Cryptococcus*) should also be considered in the differential diagnosis of multiple pulmonary nodules in a patient with HIV infection/acquired immunodeficiency syndrome (AIDS).

■ Essential Facts

- AIDS-related KS occurs principally in homosexual or bisexual men infected with human herpesvirus type 8.
- AIDS-related KS is a multicentric disease that may involve lymph nodes, the gastrointestinal tract, and the lung parenchyma in the presence of extensive mucocutaneous disease.
- Pulmonary KS is found in ~10% of patients with AIDS and in 50% of patients with cutaneous KS.
- The prevalence of pulmonary KS at postmortem examination in patients with AIDS is also high (30–50%).
- Affected patients typically have a low CD4-lymphocyte count (< 100/mm3).

- Thoracic involvement from KS includes bilateral pulmonary nodules in a peribronchovascular distribution, coalescent nodular and irregular opacities with a "flame shape" appearance, and hilar-mediastinal lymphadenopathy.
- Enhancing neck, axillary, abdominal, and pelvic lymph nodes are also common.
- Bilateral pleural effusions are common, and their presence has been associated with a poor outcome.
- Cavitary pulmonary lesions have also been reported.
- Osteolytic lesions in the sternum and thoracic spine as well as soft-tissue masses with skin and subcutaneous fat involvement are other imaging findings.

■ Other Imaging Findings

- Nuclear medicine studies with sequential thallium and gallium scanning have been used to help differentiate between KS and other diseases that affect the lungs in patients with AIDS. Gallium uptake is generally negative in KS and positive in lymphoma and infection. Thallium uptake is typically positive in lymphoma and KS. Results of testing with indium 111–labeled polyclonal human immunoglobulin are negative in KS.

✓ Pearls & ✗ Pitfalls

- ✓ The incidence of KS has declined significantly since the introduction of highly active antiretroviral therapy.
- ✗ The imaging manifestation of thoracic involvement in KS can be misleading because it can be seen as an isolated event or associated with an opportunistic infection.

Case 50

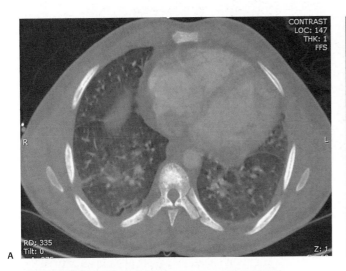

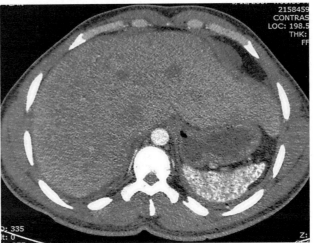

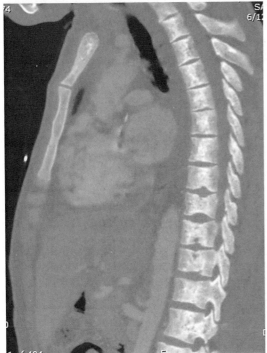

■ **Clinical Presentation**

A 23-year-old man with acute chest pain and cough. The patient had recurrent episodes of chest pain in the past.

■ Imaging Findings

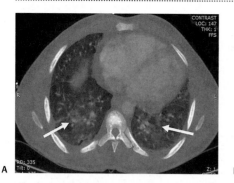
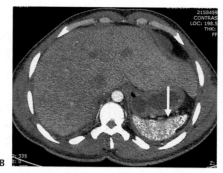
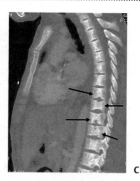

(A–C) Contrast-enhanced computed tomography of the chest: Lung window image at the level of the lower lobes shows bilateral basilar parenchymal opacities and a mild degree of cardiomegaly (*white arrows*, A). Axial image at the level of the upper abdomen shows extensive punctate calcification of the spleen (*arrow*, B). Bone window mid-thoracic sagittal reconstruction shows diffuse abnormal density of the spine with end plate deformity of the vertebral bodies (*black arrows*, C).

■ Differential Diagnosis

- *Sickle cell disease (SCD), acute chest syndrome (ACS):* ACS in patients with SCD presents with a variable degree of parenchymal opacities, which may be unilateral or bilateral.
- *SCD with pneumonia:* Patients with SCD have a high incidence of pneumonia that presents with a variable degree of parenchymal opacities.
- *SCD with pulmonary edema:* Pulmonary edema may develop in patients with SCD from a variety of causes: severe anemia, aggressive volume resuscitation, renal insufficiency from renal infarction, dilated cardiomyopathy, and pulmonary hypertension.

■ Essential Facts

- ACS is an acute pulmonary disease that develops in patients with SCD. It is one of the most common causes of hospitalization in these patients and is responsible for 25% of deaths among them.
- ACS occurs in 15 to 40% of patients with SCD and is more prevalent in children and in patients with homozygous disease.
- ACS is defined as the presence of a new pulmonary opacity on a chest radiograph in conjunction with at least one other new symptom or sign: chest pain, wheezing, cough, tachypnea, and/or fever higher than 38.5°C.
- ACS can be caused by different mechanisms in both infectious and noninfectious conditions. Infection, fat embolism, and rib infarction are the most common.
- Pulmonary embolism and in situ thrombosis in the pulmonary vasculature are other, less common causes of ACS.

- The most common infectious agents in patients with ACS/SCD are *Chlamydia pneumoniae* and *Mycoplasma pneumoniae*. Other, less common infectious agents are *Streptococcus pneumoniae* and *Haemophilus influenzae*.
- Fat emboli originate in bone marrow that becomes infarcted during acute crises. Necrotic fragments break loose and are trapped in the pulmonary vascular bed.
- Chronic lung disease develops in ~4% of patients with SCD, presumably secondary to recurrent episodes of infarction and infection. Interstitial pulmonary fibrosis, parenchymal irregular scars, pleural thickening, and bronchiectasis develop and involve predominantly the lower lobes.
- Pulmonary arteriolar intimal hyperplasia develops, resulting in pulmonary arterial hypertension.
- Bone infarcts affecting the ribs and humeral heads are also common imaging findings.
- Chronic and recurrent episodes of splenic infarction are common. The replacement of the tissue of the spleen by scar and calcification leads to a small, densely calcified, nonfunctional organ (autosplenectomy).

✓ Pearls & ✗ Pitfalls

- ✓ Infarction affecting the vertebral body end plate creates a step-off deformity known as the Reynolds sign, which is associated with concurrent overgrowth of the adjacent secondary ossification center and results in H-shaped deformity, which is considered almost pathognomonic for SCD.
- ✗ Paraspinal masses resulting from extramedullary hematopoiesis are additional imaging findings on thoracic imaging examinations and should not be confused with neoplasm or lymphadenopathy. Their nature can be confirmed by imaging with technetium 99m sulfur colloid.

Case 51

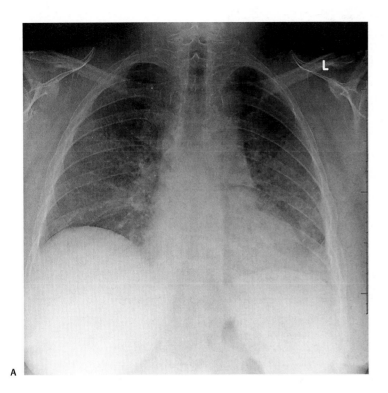

A

▪ Clinical Presentation

A 35-year-old woman who is a smoker with the gradual onset of mild dyspnea.

Further Work-up

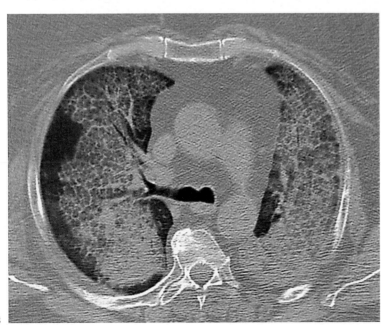

B

■ Imaging Findings

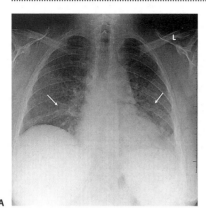
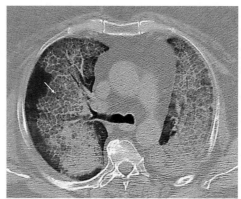

A   B

(A) Chest radiograph demonstrates central ground-glass and linear interstitial opacity bilaterally (*arrows*).
(B) Contrast-enhanced computed tomography (lung windows) shows geographic ground-glass opacity
(*arrow*), with interlobular septal thickening sharply demarcated from normal lung.

■ Differential Diagnosis

- *Pulmonary alveolar proteinosis:* The central geographic
  pattern, lack of adenopathy, and mild symptoms favor
  alveolar proteinosis.
- *Pulmonary edema:* This is typically associated with cardiomegaly and pleural effusions. The presentation is usually
  more acute.
- Pneumocystis jiroveci *pneumonia:* This typically presents
  with fever and hypoxia. Patients are immunosuppressed.
  Cysts may be present.

■ Essential Facts

- The "crazy-paving" sign represents thickened interlobular septa superimposed on a background of ground-glass
  opacity. The pattern resembles paving stones of various
  shapes.
- The crazy-paving pattern was first reported in alveolar
  proteinosis but can be seen in other diseases with air-
  space and interstitial components.
- Ground-glass opacity represents alveoli filled with phos-
  pholipid material that stains with periodic acid–Schiff.
- Nocardiosis (*Nocardia asteroides*) is the most common
  complicating superinfection.
- Pulmonary alveolar proteinosis is diagnosed and treated
  with bronchoalveolar lavage.
- Alveolar proteinosis can show uptake on gallium scan.

✓ Pearls & ✗ Pitfalls

- ✓ Crazy-paving is classic but not specific for pulmonary
  alveolar proteinosis.
- ✗ Retained lavage fluid may falsely worsen the imaging
  findings in the acute post-treatment period.
- ✗ Bronchoalveolar carcinoma can have a similar appearance but may be more focal and associated with lymphadenopathy.
- ✗ Exogenous lipoid pneumonia can manifest with the
  crazy-paving pattern. If concomitant consolidation is
  present, however, it is typically of low attenuation.

Case 52

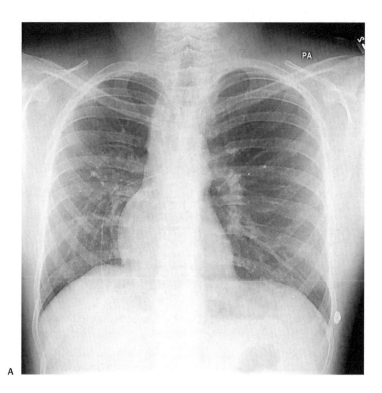

A

Clinical Presentation

An 18-year-old man with a positive purified protein derivative test result.

Further Work-up

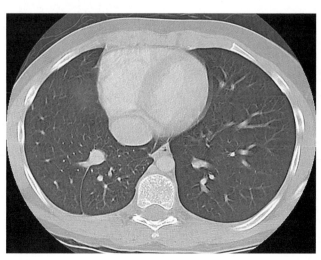

B

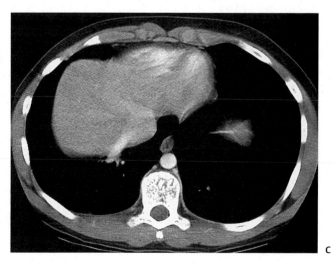

C

■ Imaging Findings

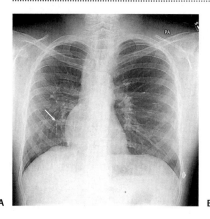
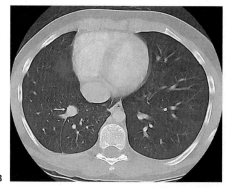
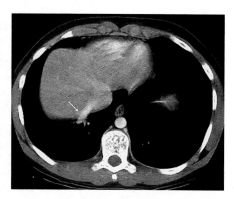

(A) Chest radiograph demonstrates a small right hemithorax with a curved linear opacity descending from the right midlung to the diaphragm (*arrow*). **(B)** Contrast-enhanced computed tomography (CT) of the chest (lung windows) demonstrates an anomalous pulmonary vein (*arrow*). **(C)** Contrast-enhanced CT of the chest (soft-tissue windows) shows the anomalous pulmonary vein draining into the inferior vena cava (IVC; *arrow*).

■ Differential Diagnosis

- **Scimitar syndrome:** The anomalous vein is right-sided and shaped like a Turkish sword (scimitar), and it drains into the IVC. The right lung is hypoplastic.
- *Swyer-James syndrome:* This is characterized by post-infectious bronchiolitis obliterans typically involving only one lung and leading to volume loss. The pulmonary venous anatomy is, however, normal.
- *Pulmonary sequestration:* This is typically seen at the left base with systemic arterial supply and normal (intralobar) or systemic (extralobar) venous drainage. A complex lung mass should be identified.

■ Essential Facts

- Scimitar syndrome is also known as hypogenetic lung syndrome and congenital pulmonary venolobar syndrome.
- It is a form of partial anomalous pulmonary venous return.
- Fifty percent of patients are asymptomatic.
- It is almost exclusively right-sided.
- The degree of pulmonary hypoplasia is variable.
- An anomalous vein typically drains into the IVC.
- The diameter of the vein typically increases as it descends.
- The draining site (typically the IVC) is usually enlarged.
- The right pulmonary artery is hypoplastic.
- Scimitar syndrome may be associated with bronchogenic cyst, horseshoe lung, or accessory diaphragm.

✓ Pearls & ✗ Pitfalls

- ✓ Twenty-five percent of patients have associated congenital heart disease, most often a sinus venosus atrial septal defect.
- ✗ There may be systemic arterial supply to the right lower lobe.
- ✗ The right pulmonary artery may enlarge when the entire right lung is drained by the anomalous vein.

Case 53

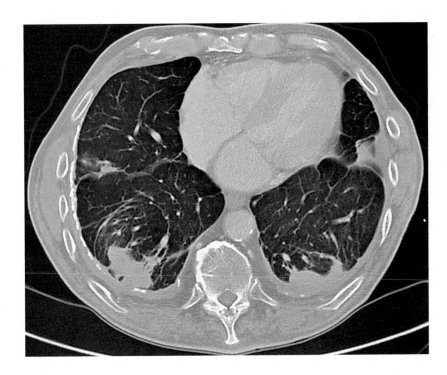

■ Clinical Presentation

A 62-year-old man with shortness of breath and a history of asbestos exposure.

■ Imaging Findings

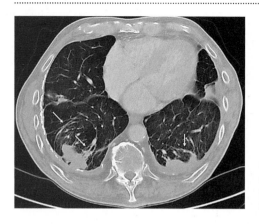

Contrast-enhanced computed tomography (lung window) through the lung bases shows bilateral pleural thickening and calcified pleural plaques. Foci of consolidation abut the posterior pleura bilaterally. Long curvilinear opacities extend from the masses anteriorly (*arrows*). The margins of the masses form an acute angle with the pleura.

■ Differential Diagnosis

• ***Rounded atelectasis:*** The presence of curvilinear opacities, the "comet tail" sign, and an association with pleural thickening make this diagnosis the top consideration.
• *Bronchogenic carcinoma:* Although this should be considered, given the patient's age, the association with pleural thickening and presence of the comet tail sign favor rounded atelectasis.
• *Mesothelioma:* Although the patient has a history of asbestos exposure, mesothelioma is rare. The mass is expected to form obtuse, not acute, angles with the visceral pleura. Mesothelioma is usually associated with a pleural effusion and hemithoracic volume loss. Bilaterality is rare.

■ Essential Facts

• Rounded atelectasis is an unusual form of atelectasis associated with extensive pleural folding and invagination.
• It abuts pleural effusion or thickening.
• Interlobular septa are thickened and fibrotic.
• Rounded atelectasis is most commonly associated with asbestos-related pleural disease but may occur with any cause of pleural fibrosis.
• It is typically found in the posterior aspect of the lower lobes.
• A swirling bronchovascular bundle is thought to resemble a comet's tail.
• An atelectatic lung may show homogeneous contrast enhancement.
• Air bronchograms are present in 60% of cases.

✓ Pearls & ✗ Pitfalls

✓ The comet tail sign helps differentiate rounded atelectasis from other masses based in the pleura.
✗ Rounded atelectasis may enlarge over time.
✗ Contrast enhancement may cause it to mimic neoplastic lesions.
✗ Fine-needle aspiration or biopsy is necessary if the imaging findings are equivocal.

Case 54

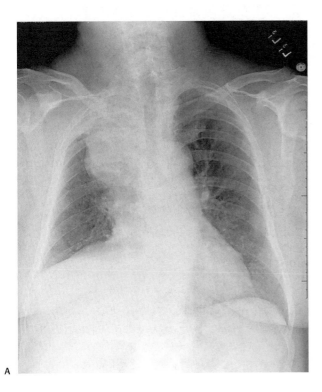

A

Clinical Presentation

A 70-year-old woman who is a smoker with chronic cough.

Further Work-up

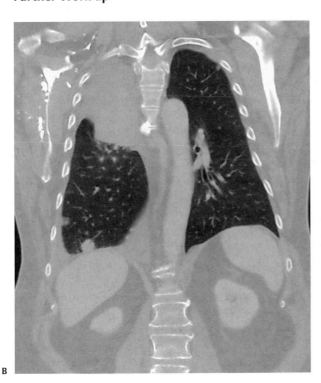

B

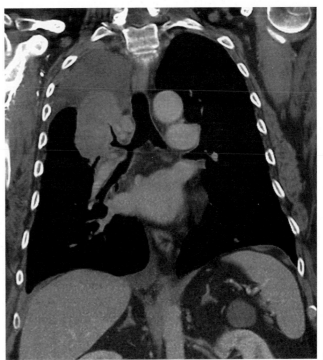

C

■ Imaging Findings

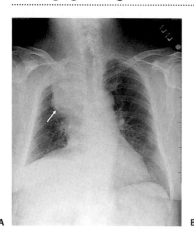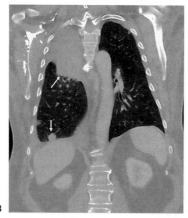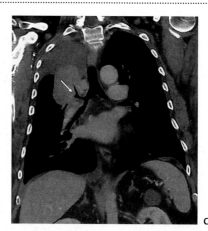

(A) Chest radiograph demonstrates right upper lobe atelectasis (*arrow*). The minor fissure is elevated and medially displaced. Proximally, however, there is convexity of the fissure. **(B)** Coronal computed tomography (CT) reconstruction (lung windows) demonstrates the right upper lobe atelectasis. A pulmonary nodule is seen at the right base that was not convincingly evident on the radiograph (*arrow*, B). **(C)** Coronal CT reconstruction (soft-tissue windows) clearly depicts a proximal mass obstructing the right upper lobe bronchus (*arrow*, C).

■ Differential Diagnosis

- ***Primary bronchogenic carcinoma:*** An obstructing central mass in an older smoker is high suggestive of primary lung carcinoma. More than 75% of primary lung carcinomas are non–small-cell lung carcinomas. The pulmonary nodule in the right lower lobe is a metastasis. Metastases are found in 50% of patients at presentation.
- *Carcinoid:* Eighty-five percent of typical carcinoids develop in the main, lobar, or segmental bronchi. There may be calcification, and intense contrast enhancement is expected. Carcinoids may present with lobar atelectasis. Although the findings may represent carcinoid, these malignancies are extremely rare in comparison with primary lung carcinomas.
- *Foreign body:* Foreign body aspiration may present with lobar atelectasis. Alternatively, the foreign body can have a "ball valve" effect, leading to lobar hyperinflation. However, the relative rarity of foreign body aspiration in the adult population and the convexity of the minor fissure centrally make this diagnosis unlikely. The CT findings of an obstructing mass and pulmonary metastasis exclude this possibility.

■ Essential Facts

- The "Golden *S*" sign is indicative of a central obstructing mass.
- Lobar atelectasis results in hemithoracic volume loss and increased lung opacity.
- When the right upper lobe collapses, the minor and major fissures shift superomedially.

- The minor fissure assumes a "reverse S" (right upper lobe) configuration when the obstructing central mass creates a convexity in the normally concave displaced fissure. It can be seen in other lobes as well.

■ Other Imaging Findings

- Juxtaphrenic peaking describes a triangular opacity projecting superiorly over the medial half of the diaphragm. It is likely due to upward retraction of the inferior accessory fissure and can also be seen with upper lobe collapse.
- The Luftsichel sign describes a hyperinflated left lower lobe filling the anteromedial left apex and creating a sharp lucency between the aorta and the opaque collapsed left upper lobe.

✓ Pearls & ✕ Pitfalls

- ✓ The bowed appearance of the minor fissure creates the Golden *S* sign and should prompt further investigation for a central obstructing mass.
- ✕ The displaced minor fissure may simulate a widened mediastinum (when parallel to the mediastinum) or an apical cap (when compressed superiorly).

Case 55

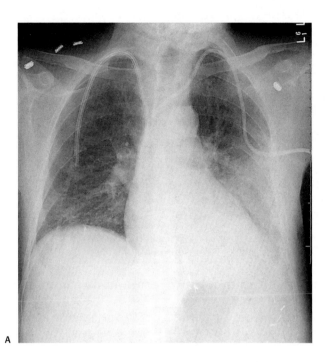

A

Clinical Presentation

A 53-year-old man with fever and shortness of breath 2 weeks after stem cell transplant.

Further Work-up

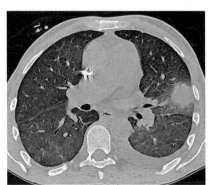

B

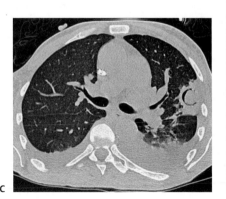

C

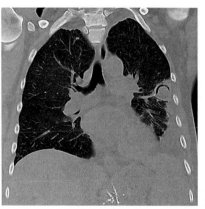

D

■ **Imaging Findings**

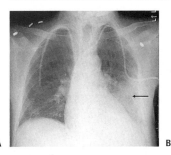 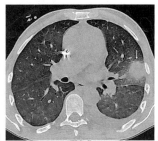 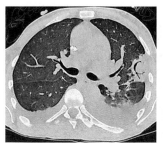 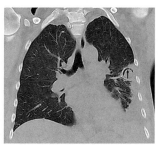

A   B   C   D

(A) Frontal chest radiograph demonstrates air-space opacity in the periphery of the left lung (*arrow*). **(B)** Noncontrast computed tomography (CT; lung window) demonstrates a solid mass in the left upper lobe with surrounding ground-glass opacity (*arrow*). There is patchy ground-glass opacity in the superior segments of the lower lobes. A left pleural effusion is present. **(C)** Noncontrast CT (lung window) obtained 1 week later demonstrates a peripheral crescentic collection of air surrounding the central solid mass (*black arrow*). The surrounding ground-glass opacity has resolved. **(D)** Noncontrast CT (coronal) shows the air crescent (*black arrow*) to advantage.

■ **Differential Diagnosis**

- *Invasive aspergillosis:* Ground-glass opacity surrounding a nodule or consolidation is usually related to hemorrhage and suggests invasive aspergillosis in neutropenic patients. The development of peripheral air represents the resorption of necrotic tissue by leukocytes and corresponds to the recovery of granulocytic function.
- *Bacterial pneumonia:* The development of cavitation and lung abscess may be seen with bacterial infections; however, the specific imaging findings and patient history in this case favor a fungal infection.
- *Pulmonary Wegener granulomatosis:* Hemorrhage due to noninfectious causes such as Wegener granulomatosis can result in the "CT halo" sign. Additionally, up to 50% of the pulmonary nodules cavitate. However, the clinical history and lack of additional nodules argue against Wegener granulomatosis.

■ **Essential Facts**

- Pulmonary aspergillosis is subdivided into four categories based on the virulence of the organisms and the patient's immune response: saprophytic (aspergilloma), hypersensitivity (allergic bronchopulmonary aspergillosis), semi-invasive (chronic necrotizing), and invasive (airway-invasive or angioinvasive).
- Angioinvasive aspergillosis occurs almost exclusively in immunocompromised patients with severe neutropenia.
- A zone of ground-glass attenuation surrounding a pulmonary nodule or consolidation is known as the CT halo sign.
- The nodule represents foci of infarction, and the halo results from alveolar hemorrhage.
- A crescent-shaped or circumferential lucency within parenchymal consolidation or a nodule is the "air crescent" sign.
- The infarcted center retracts, and leukocytes resorb the peripheral necrotic tissue. Air fills the space between the devitalized tissue and surrounding parenchyma.

- The air crescent sign develops in up to 50% of cases.
- The air crescent sign is usually seen 2 weeks after the initiation of treatment and correlates with the resolution of neutropenia.
- The CT halo sign has also been reported in infections with other fungal species, such as mucormycosis, candidiasis, and coccidioidomycosis.
- Wedge-shaped hemorrhagic infarcts based in the pleura may be seen.
- Invasion of the pleural space can result in empyema or pneumothorax.

✓ **Pearls &** ✗ **Pitfalls**

✓ In severely neutropenic patients, the CT halo and air crescent signs are highly suggestive of angioinvasive aspergillosis.

✗ An aspergilloma is seen in cases of *Aspergillus* infection without invasion. An aspergilloma is a fungus ball (mycetoma) that develops within a preexisting lung cavity.

✗ The Monad sign of aspergilloma represents the crescentic radiolucency above the gravity-dependent radiopaque lesion and should not be confused with the air crescent sign.

✗ The halo sign has also been demonstrated in hemorrhagic lung metastasis, Kaposi sarcoma, and Wegener granulomatosis.

Case 56

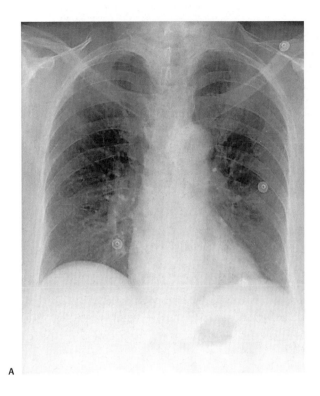

A

■ Clinical Presentation

A 43-year-old man with chest pain.

Further Work-up

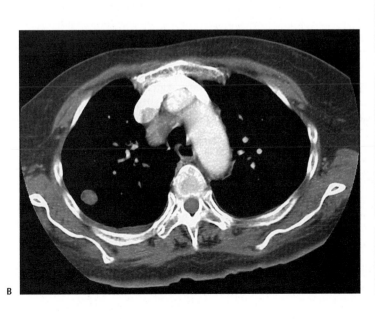

B

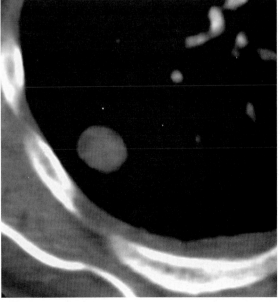

C

■ Imaging Findings

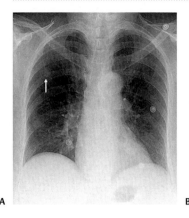
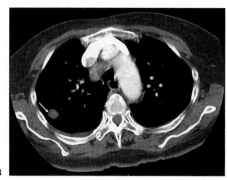
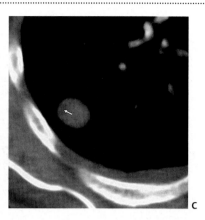

A   B   C

(A) Chest radiograph demonstrates a well-circumscribed 2-cm pulmonary nodule in the right upper lobe (*arrow*). **(B)** Contrast-enhanced computed tomography (CT) confirms a well-circumscribed solitary pulmonary nodule of heterogeneous density (*arrow*). **(C)** Magnified CT image of the nodule demonstrates a focus of macroscopic fat in its lateral aspect (*arrow*).

■ Differential Diagnosis

- ***Hamartoma:*** Fat density within a solitary pulmonary nodule is a reliable indicator of a pulmonary hamartoma.
- *Granuloma:* A postinfectious or postinflammatory granuloma is the most common cause of a solitary pulmonary nodule. Calcification is present in ~50% of granulomas. Benign patterns of calcification evident in granulomas include diffuse, central, and concentric/lamellated.
- *Primary lung carcinoma:* Nodules larger than 3 cm that have spicular, lobulated, or ill-defined margins and demonstrate growth should be aggressively investigated for their malignant potential.

■ Essential Facts

- Hamartoma is the most common benign tumor of the lung and the third most common cause of a solitary pulmonary nodule.
- Hamartoma is likely an acquired lesion resulting from the disorganized benign neoplastic proliferation of mesenchymal cells in the bronchial wall.
- Hamartomas are usually peripheral, solitary, and less than 3 cm in size.
- Up to 50% demonstrate calcification, with chondroid "popcorn" calcification virtually diagnostic.
- Intranodular fat is identified in up to 50% of hamartomas on CT. Lipomas of the lung parenchyma are rare. They are well-circumscribed and demonstrate homogeneous fat attenuation on CT.
- Most patients are asymptomatic. The peak incidence is observed in the 6th decade of life.

- Carney triad consists of (1) a pulmonary chondromatous lesion, (2) an extra-adrenal paraganglioma, and (3) an epithelioid gastric smooth-muscle tumor. It typically occurs in young women.
- Up to 20% of hamartomas are endobronchial and manifest with airway obstruction resulting in chronic cough, hemoptysis, or fever. Endobronchial hamartomas typically contain a greater proportion of fat.

✓ Pearls & ✗ Pitfalls

- ✓ The identification of intranodular fat or characteristic popcorn calcification obviates the need for biopsy or resection in asymptomatic patients.
- ✗ Liposarcoma or renal cell carcinoma metastases may produce malignant fat-containing pulmonary nodules.
- ✗ Skin lesions, nipple shadows, and osteophytes may mimic solitary pulmonary nodules on plain radiographs.
- ✗ Hamartomas may show slow growth on serial examinations.
- ✗ Lipoid pneumonia results from the chronic aspiration of mineral, animal, or vegetable oils into the lungs, leading to pneumonitis and eventually localized granulomas and fibrosis. The characteristic CT finding is dependent consolidation with fat attenuation. A "crazy-paving" appearance may be present. In contrast to those of a hamartoma, the margins of lipoid pneumonia are poorly defined.
- ✗ In patients with Carney triad, multiple pulmonary nodules may represent metastases rather than multiple pulmonary hamartomas.

Case 57

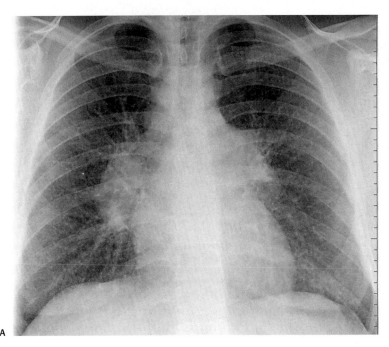
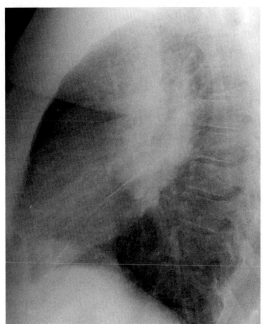

A

B

■ Clinical Presentation

A 44-year-old woman with uveitis.

Further Work-up

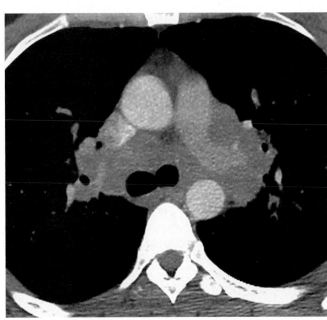

C

■ **Imaging Findings**

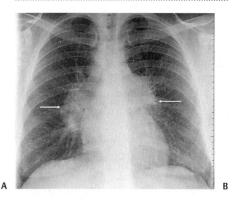
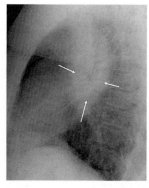
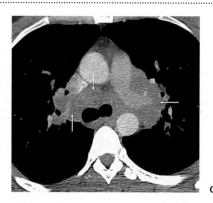

A   B   C

(A) Posteroanterior chest radiograph demonstrates symmetric hilar and right paratracheal lymphadenopathy (*arrows*). The lungs are normal. **(B)** Lateral chest radiograph shows the lymphadenopathy to advantage (*arrows*). **(C)** Computed tomography (CT) of the chest (soft-tissue windows) confirms substantial mediastinal and hilar lymphadenopathy (*arrows*).

■ **Differential Diagnosis**

- ***Sarcoidosis:*** Symmetric hilar and mediastinal lymphadenopathy in a patient with uveitis is suggestive of sarcoidosis.
- *Lymphoma:* Lymphadenopathy due to lymphoma is typically asymmetric and abuts the cardiac margins. Uveitis is not expected.
- *Tuberculosis (TB):* In primary TB, the lymphadenopathy is asymmetric and ipsilateral to the pulmonary consolidation. This patient's symptoms are not consistent with TB.

■ **Essential Facts**

- Sarcoidosis is an immunologically mediated multiple-organ granulomatous disease of unknown etiology.
- It is more common in females and African-Americans.
- It typically manifests in young and middle-aged adults.
- The clinical course and prognosis are highly variable.
- Fifty percent of patients are asymptomatic.
- Ocular involvement is present in 80% of cases.
- If the lacrimal glands are involved, lacrimal gland enlargement is typically seen bilaterally.
- Although almost any organ can be affected, intrathoracic involvement is seen in 90% of cases.
- Extrathoracic manifestations without intrathoracic disease occur in fewer than 10% of cases.
- Symmetric hilar and right paratracheal lymphadenopathy is the most common imaging finding. This is dubbed the "1, 2, 3" sign or "Garland triad." Nodes may calcify in an amorphous or eggshell pattern.
- High-resolution CT shows small perivascular nodules bilaterally, with irregular "beaded" thickening of the bronchovascular bundles and interlobular septa.
- Pulmonary involvement is typically upper lobe–predominant.
- End-stage disease results in architectural distortion, with upper lobe retraction, traction bronchiectasis, honeycombing, and cysts.

- Clinical staging can be based on the pattern of radiographic findings:
  - Stage 0: normal chest radiograph
  - Stage 1: lymphadenopathy only
  - Stage 2: lymphadenopathy and parenchymal disease
  - Stage 3: parenchymal disease only
  - Stage 4: pulmonary fibrosis
- Miliary nodules, bronchial wall thickening, and ground-glass opacity are less commonly seen.
- "Alveolar sarcoidosis" demonstrates large peripheral opacities with air bronchograms.

■ **Other Imaging Findings**

- Activity on gallium 67 scan results in the "lambda" sign, with paratracheal and hilar uptake, and the "panda" sign, with lacrimal and parotid uptake.
- Fluorodeoxyglucose uptake is variable in intensity and pattern.

✓ **Pearls & ✗ Pitfalls**

✓ Beaded interlobular septal thickening can also occur in lymphangitic carcinomatosis; however, in contrast to that seen in sarcoidosis, it is not associated with lobular architectural distortion and is unlikely to have a perihilar distribution.

✓ The combination of erythema nodosum, arthralgia, and intrathoracic lymphadenopathy is called Löfgren syndrome.

✓ The combination of fever, parotid and ocular involvement, and facial palsy is called Heerfordt syndrome.

✗ The major complications of sarcoidosis are fibrosis, cor pulmonale, and mycetoma formation.

✗ In addition to the overlap in imaging findings with lymphadenopathy, a lymphoproliferative disorder is more than five times more likely to develop in patients with sarcoidosis.

Case 58

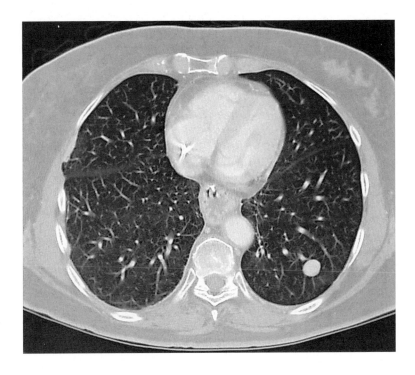

■ Clinical Presentation

A 72-year-old woman with cough.

■ Imaging Findings

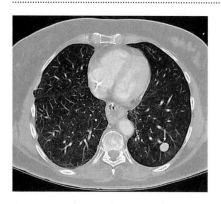

Contrast-enhanced computed tomography demonstrates a well-circumscribed 2-cm pulmonary nodule in the left lower lobe (*arrow*).

■ Differential Diagnosis

- ***Inflammatory myofibroblastic tumor:*** This most commonly presents as a solitary, peripheral, sharply circumscribed mass. The imaging features are, however, variable and nonspecific.
- *Granuloma:* A postinfectious or postinflammatory granuloma is the most common cause of a solitary pulmonary nodule. Calcification is present in ~50% of granulomas. Benign patterns of calcification evident in granulomas include diffuse, central, and concentric/lamellated.
- *Primary lung carcinoma:* Nodules larger than 3 cm that have spicular, lobulated, or ill-defined margins and demonstrate growth should be aggressively investigated for their malignant potential.

■ Essential Facts

- Inflammatory myofibroblastic tumor is a rare benign tumor with many names: inflammatory pseudotumor, plasma cell granuloma, histiocytoma, fibroxanthoma, and mast cell granuloma.
- It is the most common primary lung mass in children.
- It affects a wide age range and shows no gender predilection.
- Up to 20% of patients have an antecedent pulmonary insult.
- Calcification is uncommon but occurs more frequently in children.
- Many patients have a history of respiratory infection.
- The tumor shows a predilection for the lower lobes.
- Cavitation and lymphadenopathy are rare.

■ Other Imaging Findings

- Inflammatory myofibroblastic tumor demonstrates intermediate signal intensity on T1-weighted magnetic resonance imaging (MRI) and high signal on T2-weighted MRI.
- Multiple lesions are seen in 5% of cases.
- Intravascular, pleural-based, and endobronchial involvement has been described.

✓ Pearls & ✗ Pitfalls

- ✓ Inflammatory myofibroblastic tumor most commonly involves the lungs and orbits but has been described in nearly every site in the body.
- ✗ The majority of these tumors slowly increase in size and may invade surrounding structures.

Case 59

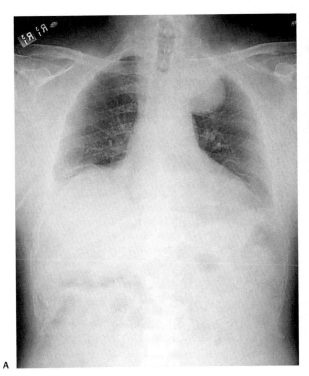

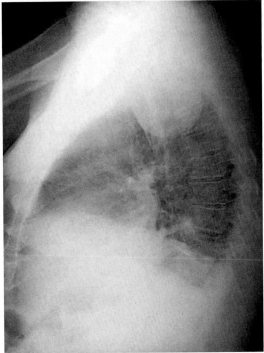

A

B

Clinical Presentation

A 50-year-old man with back pain.

Further Work-up

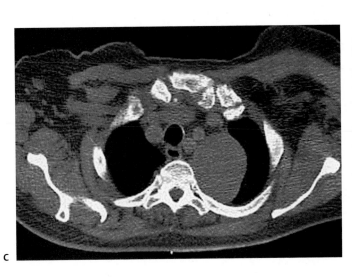

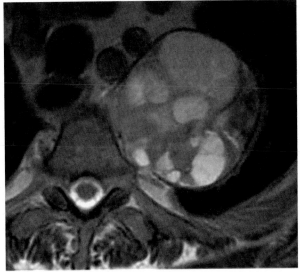

C

D

■ Imaging Findings

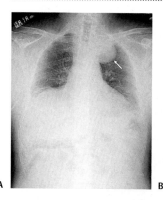
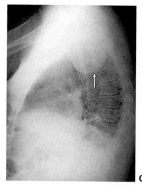
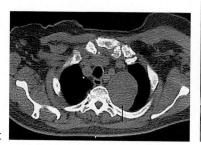
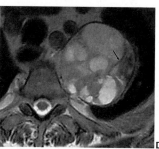

(A) Frontal chest radiograph demonstrates a large, well-circumscribed mass in the left upper chest (*arrow*). There is no evidence of rib destruction. **(B)** Lateral chest radiograph confirms the smooth inferior margin of the mass (*arrow*); however, the precise location of the abnormality cannot be determined. **(C)** Non-contrast computed tomography (soft-tissue windows) shows that the mass has heterogeneous density. It forms obtuse angles with the pleura, suggesting an extrapulmonary location (*arrow*). **(D)** T2-weighted magnetic resonance imaging (MRI) shows that the mass has heterogeneous but predominantly high signal intensity and multiple hypointense septa (*arrow*).

■ Differential Diagnosis

- ***Schwannoma:*** More than 90% of posterior mediastinal masses are neurogenic in origin. The smooth margins and signal characteristics favor a nerve sheath tumor. Cystic spaces can be intermixed within the tissue, resulting in high signal intensity on T2-weighted MRI. Adjacent osseous erosion and remodeling would be expected, however.
- *Meningocele:* A meningocele is a nonenhancing cystic mass. It should mimic the density and intensity of cerebral spinal fluid. Enlargement of the neural foramen and contiguity with the thecal sac are expected.
- *Lymphoma:* Additional intrathoracic lymphadenopathy would be expected. Signal intensity on T2-weighted MRI is variable. High signal on T2-weighted MRI may represent active disease, inflammation, cystic change, or immature fibrosis.

■ Essential Facts

- Schwannomas arise from the nerve sheath and consist of Schwann cells in a collagenous matrix.
- They are also called neurinomas or neurilemmomas.
- They have a true capsule.
- The mass is eccentric to the affected nerve.
- Schwannomas are the most common intradural extramedullary mass.
- They are typically solitary; multiple schwannomas are seen in neurofibromatosis type 2.

- When symptomatic, they usually present with pain associated with movement.
- They typically demonstrate intense enhancement.
- They often cause enlargement of the intervertebral foramen.
- Up to 15% have a dumbbell appearance, with both intra- and extradural elements.
- Calcification is seen in 10%.
- A schwannoma may be difficult to distinguish from a neurofibroma.
- Schwannomas are more likely to have a visible capsule and intratumoral cysts.
- The Carney complex consists of melanotic schwannomas, cutaneous myxomas, cardiac myxomas, and adrenal tumors.

✓ Pearls & ✗ Pitfalls

- ✓ The target sign on T2-weighted MRI (high signal intensity peripherally and low signal centrally) is seen more frequently in neurofibromas than in schwannomas.
- ✓ The visualization of fascicular bundles in neurogenic tumors is known as the fascicular sign.
- ✓ Melanotic schwannomas show high signal intensity on T1-weighted images.
- ✗ The target and fascicular signs are typically seen in benign lesions, although they have been described in malignant peripheral nerve sheath tumors.

Case 60

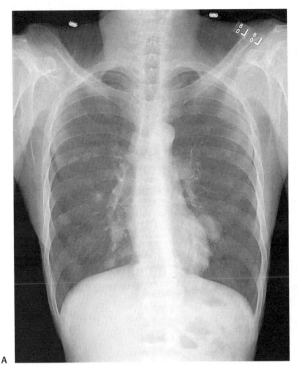

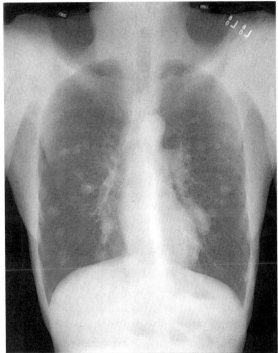

A

B

■ Clinical Presentation

A 58-year-old man with hoarseness and cough.

Further Work-up

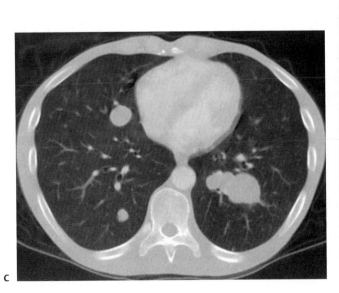

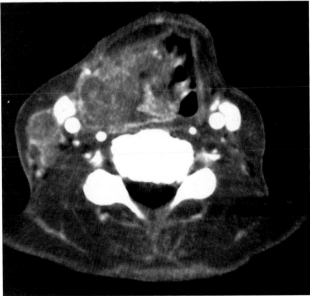

C

D

■ Imaging Findings

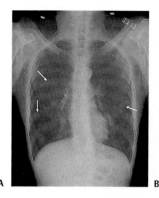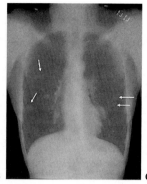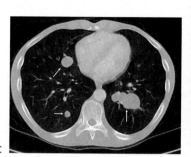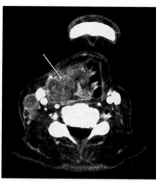

A   B   C   D

(A) Chest radiograph demonstrates multiple lower lung zone–predominant well-circumscribed pulmonary nodules (*arrows*). **(B)** Energy-subtracted chest radiograph demonstrates the pulmonary nodules to better advantage (*arrows*). **(C)** Contrast-enhanced computed tomography (CT; lung window) at the level of the coronary sinus confirms multiple well-circumscribed noncalcified pulmonary nodules (*arrows*). **(D)** Contrast-enhanced CT (soft-tissue window) at the level of the vocal cords demonstrates a large heterogeneous laryngeal mass (*arrow*) with right jugular lymphadenopathy.

■ Differential Diagnosis

- ***Pulmonary metastases of head and neck carcinoma:*** Multiple peripheral, smooth, and round pulmonary nodules in an afebrile older patient are suggestive of pulmonary metastases. The laryngeal mass and jugular lymphadenopathy make head and neck squamous cell carcinoma the most likely primary neoplasm.
- *Wegener granulomatosis:* This can demonstrate widely distributed nodules of varying size that may cavitate. Patchy, shaggy air-space opacity and pulmonary hemorrhage can also be seen. Wegener granulomatosis may also involve the trachea and cause subglottic stenosis, but typically without frank nodularity. A laryngeal mass would not be expected.
- *Granulomatous infection:* Tuberculosis, histoplasmosis, and coccidioidomycosis can result in multiple well-defined pulmonary nodules. Intrathoracic lymphadenopathy can also be seen. In the healed stage, calcification is common. In the active stage, a granulomatous infection may demonstrate consolidation and cavitation. The large laryngeal mass makes granulomatous infection unlikely.

■ Essential Facts

- Squamous cell carcinoma accounts for more than 90% of all head and neck cancers.
- Head and neck cancers account for ~3 to 5% of all cancers in the United States.
- Head and neck cancer, especially laryngeal cancer, is more common in men.
- Eighty-five percent of head and neck cancers are linked to tobacco and alcohol use.
- Human papillomavirus and Epstein-Barr virus infection, radiation, and industrial exposures have also been linked to cancers of the head and neck.
- Approximately 5% of patients with head and neck cancer have pulmonary metastases at presentation. At autopsy, 15 to 40% are found to have metastases.

- Symptoms are usually absent in patients with metastases; however, tumor bulk, airway obstruction, or pleural effusions may lead to dyspnea or cough.
- Because head and neck cancers have venous drainage directly to the lung, most metastases are disseminated by hematogenous spread.
- Hematogenous metastases usually result in multiple well-circumscribed noncalcified nodules of varying size.
- A basilar predominance is seen because of the high rate of blood flow.
- Most nodules are peripherally located.
- The "feeding vessel" sign can be seen with angiocentric nodules.
- Metastases of squamous cell carcinoma are more likely to cavitate than metastases of other cell types (4%).

✓ Pearls & ✗ Pitfalls

- ✓ Bronchopleural fistula due to subpleural cavitary metastases may result in spontaneous pneumothorax; however, this is most commonly described with metastases of osteosarcoma.
- ✓ The walls in cavitary metastases are usually thick and irregular.
- ✓ "Benign pulmonary metastases" can be seen with uterine leiomyomas or hydatidiform moles, osseous giant cell tumors, chondroblastomas, salivary pleomorphic adenomas, and meningiomas.
- ✗ Laryngotracheal papillomatosis may demonstrate laryngeal and tracheal nodularity and multiple pulmonary nodules.
- ✗ Up to 10% of all solitary pulmonary nodules are metastases.
- ✗ Given the typical patient demographics and risk factors, a solitary pulmonary nodule is more likely to be a primary lung carcinoma than a solitary metastasis in a patient with head and neck cancer.

Case 61

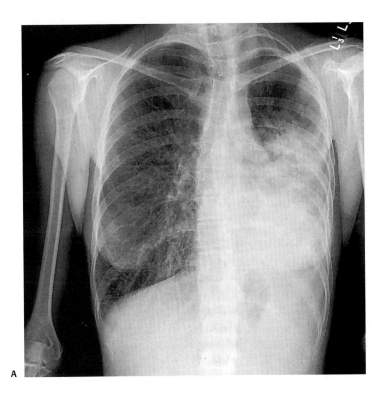

A

■ Clinical Presentation

A 78-year-old woman who is a smoker with progressive cough and dyspnea.

Further Work-up

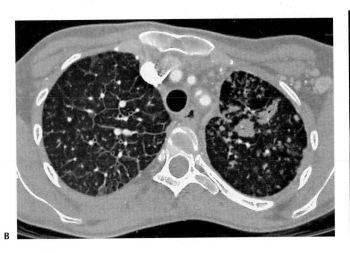

B

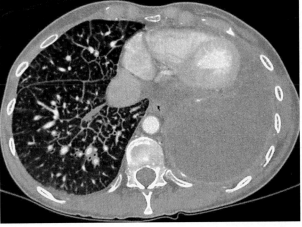

C

■ Imaging Findings

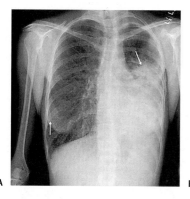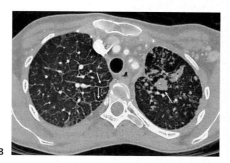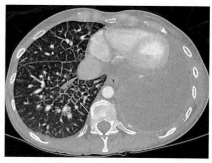

A B C

(A) Chest radiograph demonstrates a left hilar mass and large pleural effusion (*arrow*). Interlobular septal thickening is seen on the right (*arrow*). **(B)** Contrast-enhanced computed tomography (CT; lung window) at the lung apices shows multiple irregular pulmonary nodules that are predominantly centrilobular (*arrow*). There is coarse interlobular septal thickening on the right (*arrows*). **(C)** Contrast-enhanced CT (lung window) at the lung bases demonstrates a large left pleural effusion with pleural thickening and calcification. There is extensive beaded interlobular septal thickening (*arrow*). Bronchial wall thickening is also seen.

■ Differential Diagnosis

- **Lymphangitic carcinomatosis:** The patient's history, large left hilar mass with a pleural effusion, and irregular interlobular septal thickening make lymphangitic carcinomatosis the most likely diagnosis.
- *Sarcoidosis:* Nodular septal thickening can be seen with sarcoidosis. Additionally, sarcoidosis can demonstrate perilymphatic and centrilobular nodules. Lymphadenopathy would also be expected. However, the findings in this case are asymmetric and lack upper lobe predominance. Pleural effusions are uncommon with sarcoidosis. There is also no architectural distortion, which would be expected with severe sarcoidosis.
- *Pulmonary edema:* Edema typically manifests as smooth interlobular septal thickening. It is generally diffusely distributed; however, localized pulmonary edema can be seen with intrathoracic malignancy because of isolated pulmonary venous compression by a mass. Although a pleural effusion often accompanies pulmonary edema, the nodules and large left hilar mass exclude pulmonary edema as a consideration.

■ Essential Facts

- The extravasation of bloodborne tumor cells into the peribronchovascular interstitium is followed by spread along the lymphatics.
- Lung cancer may spread along the lymphatics.
- Lymphoma may enter the lymphatics retrograde via mediastinal lymph nodes.
- Lymphatic distention, interstitial pulmonary edema due to lymphatic obstruction, tumor within the interstitium, and secondary fibrotic reaction all account for the radiologic abnormalities seen within the septa and bronchovascular bundles.

- Patients present with dyspnea, cough, and reduced lung compliance and diffusing capacity.
- Lymphangitic carcinomatosis is secondary to adenocarcinomas in 80% of cases, most commonly to lung, breast, stomach, and pancreatic cancers.
- The prognosis is dismal, with a high 1-year mortality rate.
- Although the chest radiograph may be normal, septal lines, reticulonodular opacities, and subpleural edema are most commonly seen.
- Pleural effusion is seen in 60% of cases.
- Hilar and mediastinal lymphadenopathy is present in 30% of cases.
- Beaded or nodular thickening of the bronchovascular bundles, interlobular septa, and lobar fissures is best seen on high-resolution CT.
- Subpleural thickening may be evident.
- Infiltration along the centrilobular bronchovascular bundle creates a central dot within the secondary pulmonary nodule.
- The lung architecture is preserved.

✓ Pearls & ✗ Pitfalls

- ✓ If the findings are unilateral, primary lung carcinoma is the most likely diagnosis.
- ✓ A whole lobe or lung may be spared.
- ✓ Lymphangitic carcinomatosis is more common on the right.
- ✗ Drug reactions and pulmonary edema may coexist.
- ✗ Lymphoproliferative diseases such as lymphocytic interstitial pneumonia can also cause nodular interlobular septal thickening.

Case 62

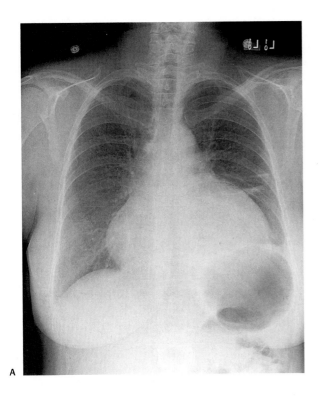

A

■ Clinical Presentation

A 50-year-old woman with dyspnea on exertion.

Further Work-up

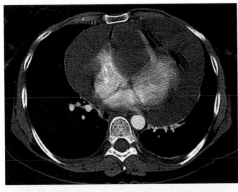

B

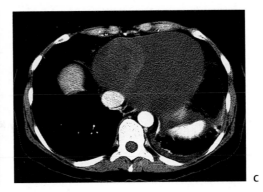

C

D

■ Imaging Findings

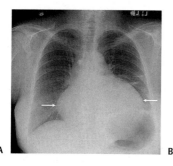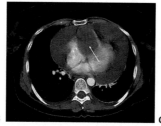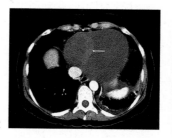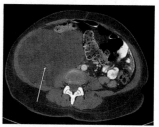

(A) Chest radiograph demonstrates a globular enlarged cardiac silhouette (*arrows*). Linear atelectasis is seen in the left lung. **(B)** Contrast-enhanced computed tomography (CT) through the right ventricle (soft-tissue window) shows a large pericardial effusion. A large mass is invading the right ventricle (*arrow*). **(C)** Contrast-enhanced CT through the caudal margin of the pericardium (soft-tissue window) shows an extensive amount of pericardial fluid. Although the fluid is predominantly of low density, a curvilinear area of high density is seen anterior to the inferior vena cava (IVC, *arrow*). **(D)** Contrast-enhanced CT (soft-tissue window) through the abdomen demonstrates a large mass occupying most of the right abdomen (*long arrow*). There is a resultant mass effect on the ascending colon and IVC. The density is heterogeneous, but there are extensive areas of very low density.

■ Differential Diagnosis

- **Cardiac metastases:** The vast majority of cardiac masses are metastatic. Associated pericardial effusion can be seen in up to 50% of patients. The large abdominal mass further supports metastases.
- *Myxoma:* Myxoma is the most common primary cardiac neoplasm. It is more commonly found in the left atrium, although 20% can be seen in the right atrium. Left atrial myxoma usually is associated with signs of pulmonary venous hypertension, mimicking mitral valve disease. Right atrial myxomas may demonstrate calcification. A myxoma would not result in a large abdominal mass.
- *Primary malignant cardiac tumor:* Angiosarcoma is the most common primary malignant tumor; however, it is far less common than metastases. Angiosarcomas are typically found in the right atrium. Myocardial and pericardial invasion can be seen. A pericardial effusion may be evident. Although metastases to the abdomen can occur, a solitary large abdominal mass would not be expected.

■ Essential Facts

- An accumulation of more than 50 mL of fluid in the pericardial space is abnormal.
- Noncardiac tumors can reach the heart by lymphatic or hematogenous dissemination, local extension, or transvenous spread.
- Primary cardiac neoplasms are up to 1000 times less prevalent than secondary neoplasms.
- Primary pericardial neoplasms are exceedingly rare and consist of pericardial teratoma in children and pericardial mesothelioma in adults.
- A pericardial effusion can manifest radiographically as a "water bottle" heart, typified by symmetric enlargement of the cardiac silhouette.

- On lateral radiograph, the "epicardial fat pad" or "Oreo cookie" sign refers to separation of the retrosternal and epicardial fat lines.
- The thickness of the normal pericardium is usually less than 2 mm.
- The most common intra-abdominal location of liposarcoma is posterior to the kidney.
- The tumors can grow to a large size before diagnosis.

■ Other Imaging Findings

- On magnetic resonance imaging, nonhemorrhagic fluid has low signal on T1-weighted spin-echo images and high signal on T2-weighted gradient-echo images.
- Hemorrhagic effusion is characterized by high signal on T1-weighted images and low intensity on T2-weighted gradient-echo images.
- Pericardial invasion is characterized by disruption, thickening, or nodularity.

✓ Pearls & ✗ Pitfalls

- ✓ A pericardial effusion in a patient with known malignancy may be a malignant pericardial effusion, or it may be secondary to radiation-induced pericarditis or drug-induced pericarditis.
- ✓ Pericardial fluid with attenuation greater than that of water suggests malignancy, hemopericardium, purulent exudate, or an effusion associated with hypothyroidism.
- ✗ Chest radiography is insensitive for detecting pericardial effusion, with roughly 200 mL fluid required to reliably make the diagnosis.
- ✗ High-grade liposarcomas may not demonstrate appreciable macroscopic fat.

Case 63

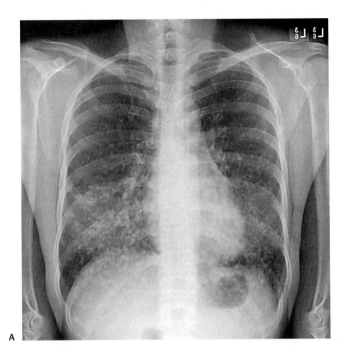

A

Clinical Presentation

A 25-year-old woman with dyspnea.

Further Work-up

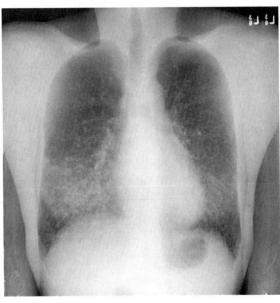

B

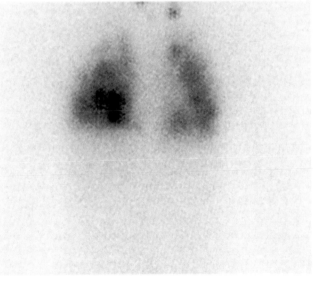

C

■ Imaging Findings

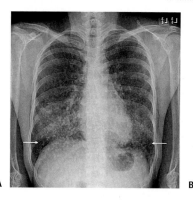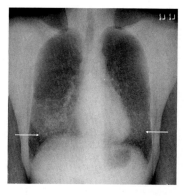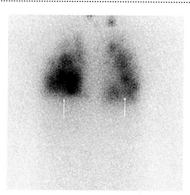

A B C

(A) Frontal chest radiograph demonstrates innumerable small, high-density pulmonary nodules that are lower lobe–predominant (*arrows*). Given their density, many of the nodules are likely calcified. **(B)** Energy-subtracted frontal chest radiograph demonstrates the nodules (*arrows*) to better advantage. **(C)** Planar anterior thoracic image from an iodine 131 (^{131}I) whole-body scan demonstrates intense lower lobe–predominant uptake (*arrows*). Uptake is also seen within the neck.

■ Differential Diagnosis

- **Metastases:** The presence of innumerable lower lobe–predominant micronodules suggests the hematogenous spread of metastases. Although the calcification of pulmonary nodules is usually suggestive of benign disease, metastatic nodules from thyroid carcinoma may calcify. Strong uptake of ^{131}I by the pulmonary nodules suggests the papillary or follicular type of thyroid cancer.
- *Granulomatous infection:* The hematogenous and endobronchial dissemination of granulomatous infection, most notably histoplasmosis, can result in multiple calcified micronodules. Although infectious signs and symptoms are expected to be present, patients may be asymptomatic. The findings on ^{131}I scan exclude granulomatous infection in this case.
- *Sarcoidosis:* The patient's age and gender make sarcoidosis a good possibility; however, pulmonary involvement is typically mid and upper lung zone–predominant. Lymphadenopathy would be expected, although parenchymal disease can occur without adenopathy in up to 20% of cases. Although dystrophic nodal involvement occurs in ~10% of cases, pulmonary calcification is exceedingly rare.

■ Essential Facts

- Papillary thyroid carcinoma is the most common type of thyroid carcinoma and carries the best prognosis.
- Hematogenous spread to the lung is seen in 4% of cases of papillary thyroid carcinoma.
- Follicular and papillary thyroid carcinomas concentrate radioactive iodine. Medullary and anaplastic carcinomas are not detected with conventional ^{131}I scintigraphy.

- Normal ^{131}I activity is seen in the choroid plexus, nasopharynx, salivary glands, thymus, stomach, bowel, bladder, and breasts. The lungs are not a normal site of ^{131}I accumulation.
- The calcification or ossification of metastatic nodules is also seen in osteosarcoma; chondrosarcoma; synovial sarcoma; giant cell tumor; adenocarcinomas of the colon, ovary, and breast; and treated choriocarcinoma.

✓ Pearls & ✗ Pitfalls

- ✓ A micronodular pattern of thyroid metastases is associated with strong ^{131}I uptake and a better prognosis, whereas macronodular lesions frequently show poor uptake.
- ✗ Radiation-induced pneumonitis and pulmonary fibrosis are rare complications of ^{131}I treatment in patients with pulmonary metastases.
- ✗ Lung opacities may persist following treatment.
- ✗ Silicosis and varicella pneumonia may present with micronodular calcifications.

Case 64

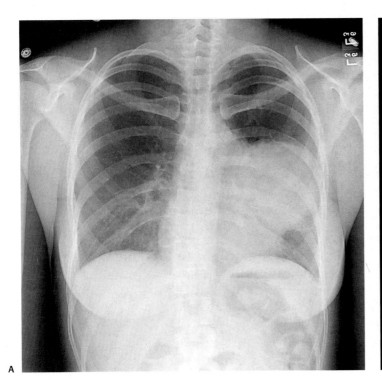

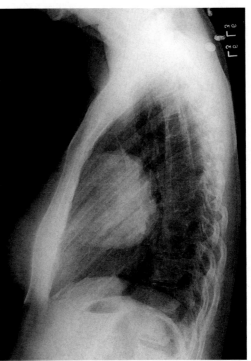

Clinical Presentation

A 30-year-old woman with fatigue.

Further Work-up

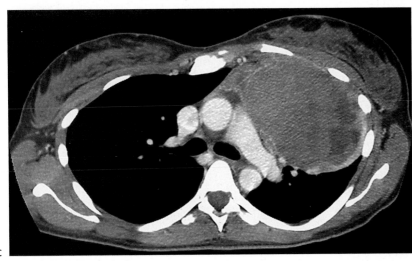

■ Imaging Findings

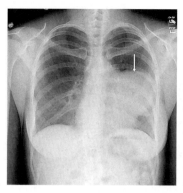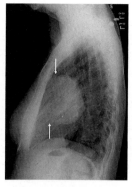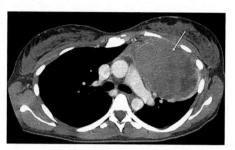

A   B   C

(A) Frontal chest radiograph demonstrates a large mass in the medial left hemithorax (*arrow*). There is loss of the left border of the heart, but the left hilar structures project through the mass (hilum overlay sign). **(B)** Lateral chest radiograph confirms the anterior location of the mass (*arrows*). **(C)** Contrast-enhanced computed tomography (CT; soft-tissue window) demonstrates a heterogeneous anterior mediastinal mass (*arrow*) that abuts the thymus.

■ Differential Diagnosis

- **Lymphoma:** A solitary noncalcified anterior mediastinal mass separate from the thymus in a patient of this age is suggestive of lymphoma. Although this patient had large B-cell non-Hodgkin lymphoma, Hodgkin disease (HD) would be the most likely diagnosis because most mediastinal lymphoma is HD.
- *Teratoma:* Mature teratomas frequently demonstrate cystic components, fat, and/or calcium. However, seminoma, the most common primary malignant germ cell tumor of the mediastinum, typically presents as a homogeneous, well-marginated soft-tissue mass in which cystic components and calcification are uncommon.
- *Castleman disease:* Also called angiofollicular or giant lymph node hyperplasia, this is more typically a middle mediastinal and hilar mass with multiple enlarged lymph nodes that may show intense enhancement. Calcification is seen in 10%.

■ Essential Facts

- Lymphoma may present with cough or chest pain.
- Weight loss, fever, and night sweats comprise "B symptoms."
- Mediastinal lymphoma is more likely to be HD than non-Hodgkin lymphoma.
- HD has a bimodal age distribution, and intrathoracic involvement is seen in 85% of cases.
- Nodular sclerosing HD is the most common subtype of HD, and there is a strong predilection for the anterior mediastinum.
- Intrathoracic involvement is seen in 50% of cases of non-Hodgkin lymphoma.
- Non-Hodgkin lymphoma commonly presents with bulky, asymmetric mediastinal and hilar lymphadenopathy.
- Diffuse large B-cell lymphoma is seen in young women.

- Calcification is rarely seen before treatment.
- Post-transplant lymphoproliferative disorder occurs in 5% of patients with solid organ transplants. The peak incidence is at 3 to 4 months after treatment. Most cases are B-cell non-Hodgkin lymphoma.
- Mild enhancement is seen on CT and magnetic resonance imaging (MRI).
- Involvement of the pleura, pericardium, and lung parenchyma is rare.

■ Other Imaging Findings

- The signal intensity on T1-weighted MRI is similar to that of muscle.
- Low signal intensity on T2-weighted MRI is seen in successfully treated lesions.
- High signal intensity on T2-weighted MRI may represent active disease, inflammation, cystic change, or immature fibrosis.
- Gallium 67 scintigraphy is useful in differentiating residual disease from posttreatment fibrosis.

✓ Pearls & ✗ Pitfalls

- ✓ When the normal hilar structures project through a mass (hilum overlay sign), the location of the mass is assumed to be anterior or posterior to the hilum.
- ✓ On posteroanterior radiograph, when the cephalic border of a mediastinal mass is obscured at or below the clavicles, the mass is located in the anterior mediastinum (cervicothoracic sign). If there is clear delineation of all borders of the mass above the clavicles, the mass is posterior to the trachea.
- ✓ Lymphoma is more likely to displace mediastinal structures than to invade them.
- ✗ Following radiation therapy, up to 20% of cases show calcification.

Case 65

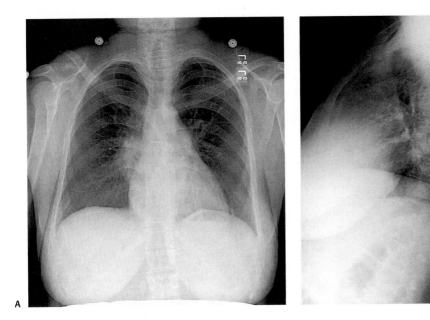

A

B

Clinical Presentation

A 32-year-old woman with chest pain.

Further Work-up

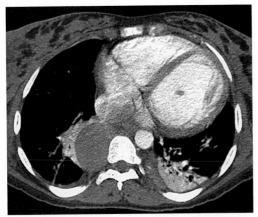

C

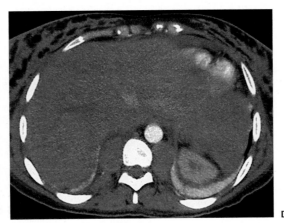

D

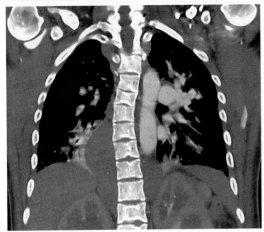

E

■ Imaging Findings

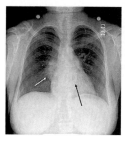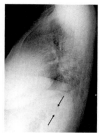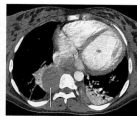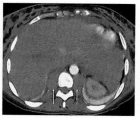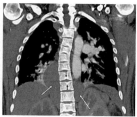

A–E

(A) Frontal chest radiograph demonstrates a right paraspinal mass with abnormal convexity of the upper azygoesophageal and right paraspinal lines (*white arrow*). The left paraspinal line is also effaced, although the lateral margin of the aorta is still seen (*black arrow*). There is mild cardiomegaly and basilar atelectasis. **(B)** Lateral chest radiograph confirms the posterior location of the mass (*arrows*). There is also multilevel vertebral end plate depression, creating "H-type" vertebrae. **(C)** Contrast-enhanced computed tomography (CT; soft-tissue window) through the level of the heart confirms a right paraspinal mass with adjacent atelectasis (*arrow*). The mass has homogeneously low attenuation. There is no evidence of osseous erosion. A much smaller lesion is seen on the left. **(D)** Contrast-enhanced CT (soft-tissue window) through the upper abdomen shows bilateral hypodense paraspinal masses (*arrows*). The lesions have smooth borders, and there is no associated osseous erosion. Hepatomegaly is present, but the spleen is not seen. **(E)** Coronal CT shows the paraspinal masses (*white arrows*) and vertebral body abnormalities (*black arrows*) to better advantage. There is also sclerosis of the left humeral head.

■ Differential Diagnosis

- **Extramedullary hematopoiesis:** Cardiomegaly, lack of visualization of the spleen, and characteristic osseous abnormalities in a patient of this age suggest underlying sickle cell anemia. In this patient, the multiple paraspinal masses likely represent extramedullary hematopoiesis.
- *Neurogenic tumor:* Neurogenic tumor is the most common cause of a posterior mediastinal mass. However, in this case, there are multiple, bilateral masses, and the lesions span multiple vertebral body levels. The axis of the lesions is vertical rather than horizontal. There is no evidence of neural foraminal involvement. The osseous findings in this case would not be expected.
- *Lymphoma:* Posterior mediastinal lymph node involvement is seen in up to 10% of patients with lymphoma. Lymphadenopathy would be expected in other locations as well. The osseous findings seen in this case would not be expected.

■ Essential Facts

- Extramedullary hematopoiesis is the proliferation of hematopoietic cells outside the bone marrow in response to marrow dysfunction.
- It is most commonly seen in patients with anemias, such as thalassemia and sickle cell anemia, and with marrow replacement diseases, such as myelofibrosis and chronic myelogenous leukemia.
- It may be due to the extrusion of marrow through vertebral cortical defects, the growth of pluripotent stem cells, or embolic phenomena from other areas of hematopoiesis.
- The liver, spleen, kidneys, lymph nodes, and posterior mediastinum are the most common sites.
- It is most commonly asymptomatic, with no treatment required, although rare cases of spinal cord compression and massive hemorrhage have been reported.
- Extramedullary hematopoiesis typically manifests as bilateral lower thoracic paraspinal masses with smooth margins.

- The masses may be confluent with abdominal paraspinal foci of extramedullary hematopoiesis.
- Calcification is uncommon.
- The masses usually contain fat.
- They may show inhomogeneous contrast enhancement.
- The condition may also manifest as masses at expanded anterior rib ends.
- Involvement of the pulmonary interstitium can manifest as a nonspecific interstitial abnormality and result in respiratory failure.

■ Other Imaging Findings

- Magnetic resonance imaging (MRI) demonstrates signal intensity similar to that of normal intramedullary hematopoietic tissue.
- T1-weighted MRI may show a rim of high signal intensity surrounding the masses. This is due to the presence of fat.
- Extramedullary hematopoiesis may show uptake on technetium 99m sulfur colloid imaging.

✓ Pearls & ✗ Pitfalls

✓ Associated hepatosplenomegaly may be seen, but the spleen will be small in sickle cell disease.

✓ The masses may regress following blood transfusion, radiation therapy, hydroxyurea therapy, or splenectomy (in patients with hereditary spherocytosis). There is a high incidence of recurrence following surgical resection.

✗ Sympathetic ganglion tumors can assume an oval shape and vertical axis and span multiple vertebral bodies, mimicking extramedullary hematopoiesis. Associated osseous erosion or a paraneoplastic syndrome may help differentiate the two entities.

✗ Large posterior mediastinal masses can be seen in Castleman disease; however, they are frequently calcified and demonstrate intense enhancement.

Case 66

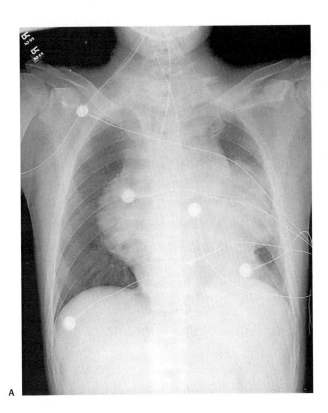

A

■ Clinical Presentation

A 30-year-old man with respiratory distress.

Further Work-up

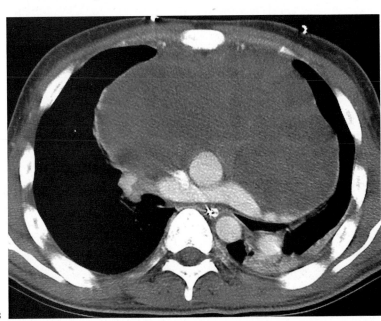

B

■ Imaging Findings

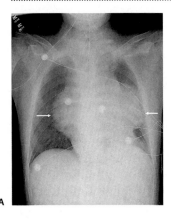
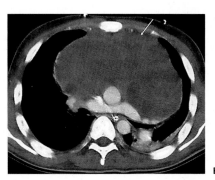

A   B

(A) Chest radiograph demonstrates an intubated patient with a large chest mass (*arrows*). Its borders with the cardiomediastinal silhouette suggest an anterior mediastinal location. There are no vertebral body or rib abnormalities. **(B)** Contrast-enhanced computed tomography of the chest (soft-tissue windows) confirms that the mass is located in the anterior mediastinum (*arrow*). Although most of the mass is smoothly marginated, there is a suggestion of local invasion involving the superior vena cava and aorta. The mass causes significant posterior displacement of the mediastinal structures, and the superior vena cava is severely attenuated.

■ Differential Diagnosis

- **Seminoma:** Seminoma presents as a bulky midline homogeneous mass of the anterior mediastinum. The patient's age and gender support the diagnosis of seminoma.
- *Thymoma:* This is a smoothly marginated mass of the anterior mediastinum. It often occurs in older patients and is associated with paraneoplastic syndromes in 40%.
- *Lymphoma:* Involvement of other lymph node groups is common. Enhancement may be heterogeneous. Systemic clinical symptoms may be present.

■ Essential Facts

- Seminoma is also known as germinoma or dysgerminoma.
- It is the most common primary malignant germ cell tumor of the mediastinum.
- Ninety percent occur in males in the 2nd, 3rd, or 4th decade of life.
- In children, malignant germ cell tumors occur in equal frequency in boys and girls.
- Most symptoms are due to mass effect.
- Serum levels of human chorionic gonadotropin and lactic dehydrogenase may be elevated.

- The tumor is large and coarsely lobulated.
- It is usually homogeneous, with soft-tissue attenuation and only mild contrast enhancement.
- Extension into the middle mediastinum can occur.
- Calcification is uncommon. Nodal calcification can be seen after treatment.
- Germinomas are highly radiosensitive, and the long-term prognosis for patients with a pure seminoma is good.
- Superior vena cava obstruction is seen in 10% of cases.
- Aortic or pulmonary artery compression can also occur.

✓ Pearls & ✗ Pitfalls

- ✓ The presence of elevated α-fetoprotein levels suggests malignant nonseminomatous elements.
- ✗ Necrosis and cystic change are seen in rare cases and may mimic a multilocular thymic cyst.

Case 67

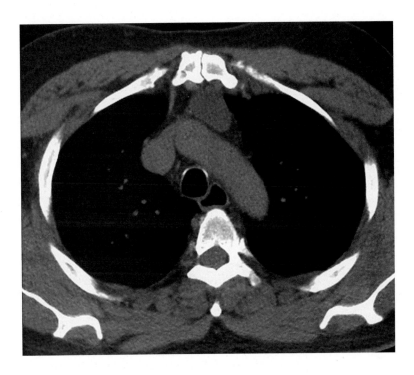

■ Clinical Presentation

A 49-year-old woman with muscle weakness.

■ Imaging Findings

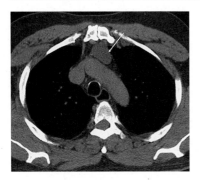

Computed tomography (CT) of the chest (soft-tissue window) demonstrates a well-circumscribed, smooth, hypodense mass in the anterior mediastinum (*arrow*). There is no evidence of vascular or pleural involvement.

■ Differential Diagnosis

- **Thymoma:** This is the most common anterior mediastinal mass, especially in patients older than 40 years of age. The homogeneous density, smooth borders, and lack of local invasion support thymoma. The clinical history suggests the presence of myasthenia gravis.
- *Germ cell tumor:* This is typically seen in younger patients. Seminomas are the most common primary malignant germ cell tumor of the mediastinum and tend to be well defined and homogeneous. Nonseminomatous germ cell neoplasms are often heterogeneous. Fat or calcium is often seen in teratomas.
- *Thymic carcinoma:* Although the age at presentation is similar to that of thymoma, paraneoplastic syndromes are uncommon. The cell types are identical to those of primary lung carcinoma. The tumors are typically heterogeneous and lobulated with poorly defined borders. Calcification is seen in up to 40%. Local invasion and lymphadenopathy may be present.

■ Essential Facts

- Thymoma is the most common primary thymic neoplasm.
- Most patients are asymptomatic, although 30% present with symptoms of compression or invasion and 40% have a paraneoplastic syndrome.
- Thymoma is associated with myasthenia gravis, pure red cell aplasia, and hypogammaglobulinemia.
- Of all patients with thymoma, 35% have myasthenia gravis.
- Of all patients with myasthenia gravis, only 15% have thymomas. Eighty-five percent of patients with myasthenia gravis have follicular thymic hyperplasia.
- The chest radiograph is normal in 25%. The mass may be seen only on lateral view.
- On CT, the mass is well defined and homogeneous.
- Approximately one-third have calcification that can be peripheral or central but is most often thin.

- Invasive thymomas are histologically identical to encapsulated thymomas but demonstrate growth outside the capsule.
- Invasive thymoma is a separate entity from thymic carcinoma, which is a histologically malignant neoplasm.

■ Other Imaging Findings

- Magnetic resonance imaging demonstrates intermediate signal on T1-weighted sequences and increased signal on T2-weighted sequences. Enhancement may be heterogeneous, with the demonstration of fibrous septa and cystic areas.

✓ Pearls & ✗ Pitfalls

- ✓ Adjacent mediastinal lymphadenopathy is rare in cases of thymoma and suggests a malignant mediastinal neoplasm, lymphoma, or metastases.
- ✗ Larger lesions may show heterogeneous enhancement and cystic areas.
- ✗ Invasive thymoma may manifest as pleural thickening or nodularity, mimicking mesothelioma or metastatic adenocarcinoma.
- ✗ Young patients may have residual thymic tissue appearing as soft-tissue nodules or attenuation in the anterior mediastinal fat. Convex borders favor a thymoma.

Case 68

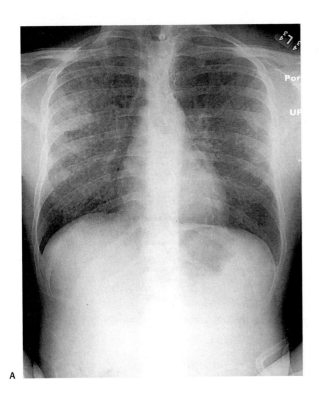

A

▪ Clinical Presentation

A 38-year-old woman with dyspnea.

Further Work-up

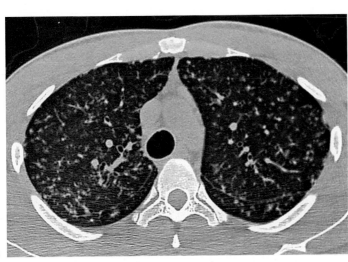

B

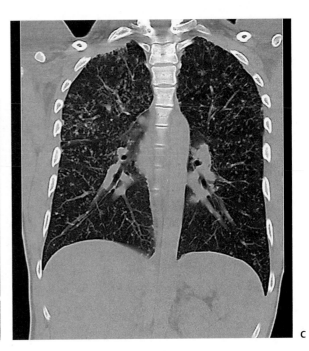

C

■ Imaging Findings

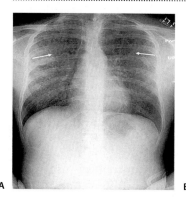
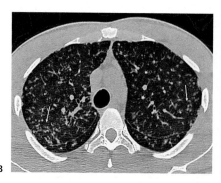
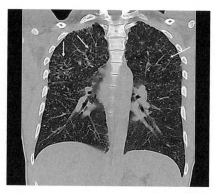

(A) Chest radiograph demonstrates upper lobe–predominant reticulonodular interstitial abnormality (*arrows*). There is no significant lymphadenopathy. **(B)** Computed tomography (CT) of the chest (lung windows) shows perilymphatic nodules and beading of the fissures. There is thickening of the bronchovascular bundles (*arrows*). **(C)** CT of the chest (coronal lung windows) shows the upper lobe distribution to advantage (*arrows*).

■ Differential Diagnosis

- **Sarcoidosis:** Upper lobe–predominant nodules in a perilymphatic distribution are suggestive of sarcoidosis.
- *Hypersensitivity pneumonitis (HP):* HP also demonstrates relative basal sparing; however, the nodules are classically centrilobular, and more ground-glass opacity is expected. An appropriate history of exposure is sometimes present.
- *Respiratory bronchiolitis:* Asymptomatic, upper lung–predominant, centrilobular nodules associated with heavy cigarette smoking are indicative of this diagnosis.

■ Essential Facts

- Sarcoidosis is an immunologically mediated multiple-organ granulomatous disease of unknown etiology.
- It is more common in females and African-Americans.
- It typically manifests in young and middle-aged adults.
- The clinical course and prognosis are highly variable.
- Fifty percent of patients are asymptomatic.
- Although almost any organ can be affected, intrathoracic involvement is seen in 90% of cases.
- Extrathoracic manifestations without intrathoracic disease occur in fewer than 10% of cases.
- Symmetric hilar and right paratracheal lymphadenopathy is the most common imaging finding. This is dubbed the "1, 2, 3" sign or "Garland triad." Nodes may calcify in an amorphous or eggshell pattern.
- High-resolution CT (HRCT) shows bilateral small perivascular nodules, with irregular "beaded" thickening of the bronchovascular bundles and interlobular septa.
- The perilymphatic distribution is evident in the peribronchovascular and subpleural interstitium as well as the interlobular septa.
- Although the granulomas are at a microscopic level, they coalesce to form visible macroscopic nodules several millimeters or more in diameter.
- Pulmonary involvement is typically upper lobe–predominant.

- Although pulmonary involvement is usually accompanied by lymphadenopathy, it can occur in isolation.
- End-stage disease results in architectural distortion, with upper lobe retraction, traction bronchiectasis, honeycombing, and cysts.
- Miliary nodules, bronchial wall thickening, and ground-glass opacity are less commonly seen.
- "Alveolar sarcoidosis" demonstrates large peripheral opacities with air bronchograms.

■ Other Imaging Findings

- Activity on gallium 67 scan results in the "lambda" sign, with paratracheal and hilar uptake, and the "panda" sign, with lacrimal and parotid uptake.
- Fluorodeoxyglucose uptake is variable in intensity and pattern.

✓ Pearls & ✗ Pitfalls

- ✓ Beading of the fissures helps differentiate perilymphatic nodules from centrilobular nodules.
- ✓ Beaded interlobular septal thickening can also occur in lymphangitic carcinomatosis, but in contrast to that seen in sarcoidosis, it is not associated with lobular architectural distortion and is unlikely to have a perihilar distribution.
- ✓ The combination of erythema nodosum, arthralgia, and intrathoracic lymphadenopathy is call Löfgren syndrome.
- ✗ Berylliosis and silicosis may have a similar appearance on imaging.
- ✗ HRCT may reveal nodules not visible by radiography in 80% of cases.
- ✗ The major complications of sarcoidosis are fibrosis, cor pulmonale, and mycetoma formation.
- ✗ In addition to the overlap in imaging findings with lymphadenopathy, a lymphoproliferative disorder is more than five times more likely to develop in patients with sarcoidosis.

Case 69

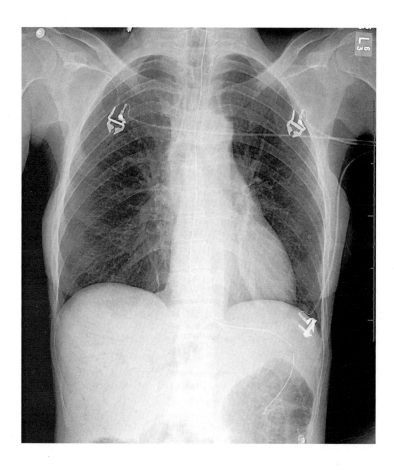

■ **Clinical Presentation**

A 38-year-old woman with sepsis.

■ Imaging Findings

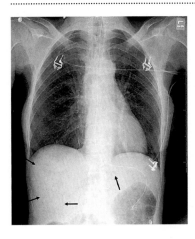

Chest radiograph demonstrates branching linear lucencies in the liver, dilated bowel loops, and pneumatosis intestinalis (*arrows*). The lungs are normal.

■ Differential Diagnosis

- **Portal venous gas:** Branching linear lucencies are usually first seen in the periphery of the liver, although in this case nearly the entire portal system is affected. The gas originates in the bowel and travels through the mesenteric veins into the portal system.
- *Pneumobilia:* This is mostly a result of a previous biliary intervention, although it can be seen with biliary enteric fistulas or cholangitis caused by a gas-forming organism. The gas is typically centrally located. Associated pneumatosis intestinalis would not be expected.

■ Essential Facts

- Portal venous gas is traditionally interpreted as an ominous sign requiring emergent surgical exploration.
- With improved imaging techniques, portal venous gas is seen more commonly and in association with several benign conditions.
- Intestinal wall pathology due to ischemia or inflammation allows intraluminal air to pass into intestinal venules.
- Severe bowel distention may also cause mucosal disruption.
- Obstructive pulmonary disease and steroid therapy have been associated with portal venous gas.

■ Other Imaging Findings

- Sonography allows the detection of small amounts of gas manifesting as hyperechoic foci throughout the portal system and parenchyma.
- On Doppler interrogation, tall, sharp, bidirectional spikes are seen.

✓ Pearls & ✗ Pitfalls

- ✓ Air is often first localized to the left lobe of the liver, which lies anteriorly.
- ✓ Gas in mesenteric venous branches is seen in a linear configuration along the mesenteric border.
- ✓ Although it can have many benign and iatrogenic causes, portal venous gas in the setting of suspected mesenteric ischemia requires surgical exploration.
- ✗ A substantial amount of portal venous gas is necessary before it can be detected on radiographs.
- ✗ Portal venous gas must be differentiated from pneumobilia, which is typically central and does not extend to the liver capsule.

Case 70

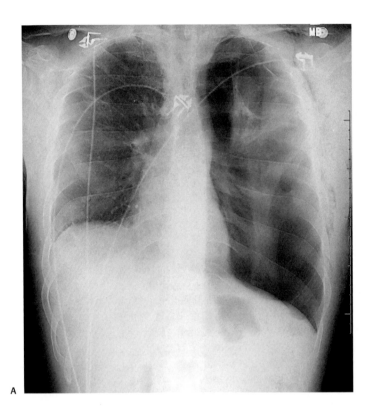

A

Clinical Presentation

A 52-year-old man with chest pain and hypotension.

Further Work-up

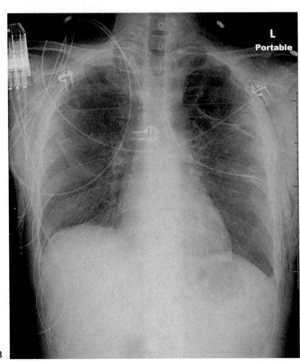

B

■ Imaging Findings

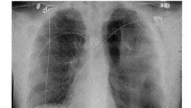
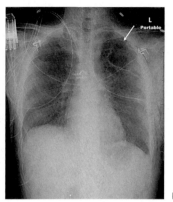

A

B

(A) Portable chest radiograph demonstrates hyperlucency of the left hemithorax with rightward mediastinal shift *(arrow)*. There is flattening of the left diaphragm and increased space between the ribs. The left pleural line is well seen, although there are multiple pleural adhesions. Subcutaneous emphysema is present on the left. **(B)** Following placement of a chest tube, the left lung has expanded and the mediastinal shift has resolved. There is minimal residual pneumothorax, as evidenced by the pleural line seen at the apex of the left lung *(arrow)*. Note the underlying emphysema and bullous changes.

■ Differential Diagnosis

- **Tension pneumothorax:** Visualization of the visceral pleural line, mediastinal shift, and hemodynamic compromise are compatible with tension pneumothorax.
- *Bullous emphysema:* Although large bullae may mimic a pneumothorax, the visceral pleural line should not be seen. The significant asymmetry would not be expected.
- *Artifact:* Skin folds, external devices, and osseous margins such as those of the scapula can mimic a pneumothorax, but the multitude of additional findings seen in this case would not be expected.

■ Essential Facts

- Tension pneumothorax results when injured tissue forms a one-way valve allowing the accumulation of air under pressure in the pleural space.
- It is most commonly due to trauma or an iatrogenic cause, especially in the setting of positive-pressure ventilation.
- Emergent needle or tube thoracostomy is required.
- After placement of a chest tube, follow-up radiography is required to confirm tube positioning and lung re-expansion.
- Lung markings should not project beyond the suspected thin pleural line.
- On supine radiographs, the air may not be seen at the lung apex and may first manifest with a deep costophrenic sulcus.
- Expiratory radiographs may increase sensitivity, although they are seldom necessary.

■ Other Imaging Findings

- Focused abdominal sonography for trauma may show a lung point, absent lung sliding, or absent "comet tail" artifact. Although some studies have shown promising accuracy, ultrasound should be considered experimental for the diagnosis of pneumothorax in an emergent setting.
- Pneumothorax ex vacuo results from acute lobar collapse. The subsequently increased negative intrapleural pressure allows gas to enter the pleural space. The seal between the visceral and parietal pleura is intact. The treatment is to relieve the bronchial obstruction rather than to place a chest tube.

✓ Pearls & ✗ Pitfalls

✓ A unilateral injury resulting in bilateral pneumothorax suggests a buffalo chest. Buffalo have one common pleural space for both lungs.

✓ A persistent air leak is suggestive of bronchopleural fistula.

✗ Although an estimate of the size of a pneumothorax (based on the separation of the lung and chest wall, or the percentage of hemithorax that is vacant) may aid in describing the radiographic findings, it is primarily the patient's clinical presentation that dictates the need to place a chest tube.

✗ Rotation of the patient on radiography may mimic mediastinal shift.

✗ Beware of skin folds, support lines, or the medial scapular margin, which may mimic a pleural line. These are better described as edges than as lines, and they often extend outside the chest wall.

✗ Re-expansion pulmonary edema may develop after placement of a chest tube.

Case 71

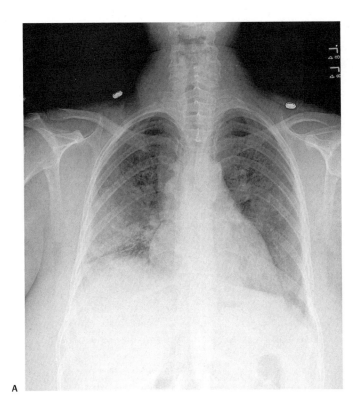

A

■ Clinical Presentation

A 44-year-old woman with hemoptysis and hematuria.

Further Work-up

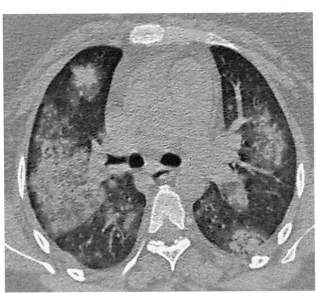

B

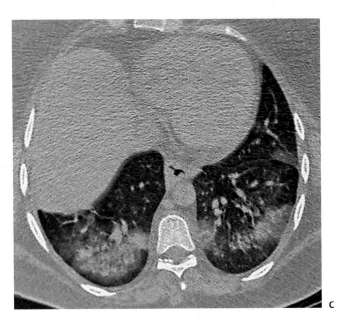

C

■ Imaging Findings

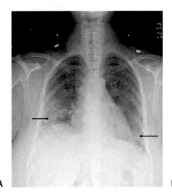
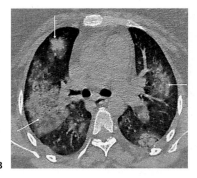
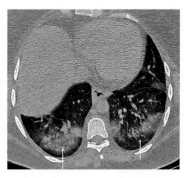

A   B   C

(A) Chest radiograph demonstrates patchy, lower lobe–predominant air-space opacity (*black arrows*). **(B)** Computed tomography (CT) of the chest (lung windows) at the level of the carina confirms multifocal ground-glass opacity (*left arrow, posterior right arrow*) with discrete nodules in the anterior right upper lobe and superior segment of the left lower lobe. The nodule in the right upper lobe has a ground-glass halo (*anterior arrow*). The nodule in the left lower lobe is cavitary. **(C)** CT of the chest (lung windows) at the lung bases (*arrows*) shows additional lower lobe consolidation and ground-glass opacity. There is no evidence of pleural or pericardial effusion, and the heart size is normal.

■ Differential Diagnosis

- **Wegener granulomatosis:** Multifocal air-space opacities and discrete pulmonary nodules demonstrating cavitation or halos in conjunction with hemoptysis and hematuria are highly suggestive of Wegener granulomatosis.
- *Churg-Strauss syndrome:* This is a pulmonary renal syndrome seen in asthmatic patients. It is associated with peripheral blood eosinophilia. As opposed to patients with Wegener granulomatosis, those with Churg-Strauss syndrome have serologic positivity for protoplasmic-staining antineutrophil cytoplasmic antibodies (p-ANCA) rather than classic antineutrophil cytoplasmic antibodies (c-ANCA); they also have a much higher frequency of cardiac involvement. Multifocal consolidation and nodules are seen. Nodules are smaller than in Wegener granulomatosis, and cavitation is rare. Pleural effusions are seen in up to one-third of cases.
- *Fungal pneumonia:* The "CT halo" sign is associated with invasive aspergillosis and represents surrounding hemorrhage. However, this sign is nonspecific and has been described in other entities, such as Wegener granulomatosis. Fungal pneumonias typically occur in immunocompromised patients.

■ Essential Facts

- Wegener granulomatosis is one of five distinct clinical syndromes of pulmonary angiitis and granulomatosis. (The others are lymphomatoid granulomatosis, necrotizing sarcoid granulomatosis, bronchocentric granulomatosis, and Churg-Strauss syndrome.)
- The classic triad consists of pulmonary disease, febrile sinusitis, and glomerulonephritis.
- c-ANCA positivity is sensitive and specific for active disease.

- Treatment with steroids and cyclophosphamide has a significant effect, although it places the patient at risk for bone marrow suppression, superimposed infection, and hemorrhagic cystitis.
- Imaging demonstrates multiple nodules that may be poorly defined because of surrounding hemorrhage.
- Cavitation develops in 50% of the nodules; the walls are usually thick and irregular initially.
- Diffuse air-space opacity is a result of hemorrhage.
- A ground-glass halo surrounding the nodule is the CT halo sign.
- Airway involvement can manifest as focal or elongated segments of stenosis, soft-tissue masses or thickening, and/or atelectasis.
- Pleural and pericardial effusions can be seen but are uncommon.
- Lymphadenopathy is not expected.
- Sinus disease manifests as a soft-tissue mass with septal and nonseptal osseous destruction.

✓ Pearls & ✗ Pitfalls

- ✓ Rapid enlargement of a nodule suggests hemorrhage or superimposed infection.
- ✓ Unlike pulmonary parenchymal lesions, airway lesions do not usually respond to medical therapy, and stenting may be required.
- ✓ The nodules may be closely associated with feeding pulmonary arteries.
- ✗ In pediatric patients, consolidation is more common than nodularity.
- ✗ Upper airway stenosis is often overlooked on radiographs.

Case 72

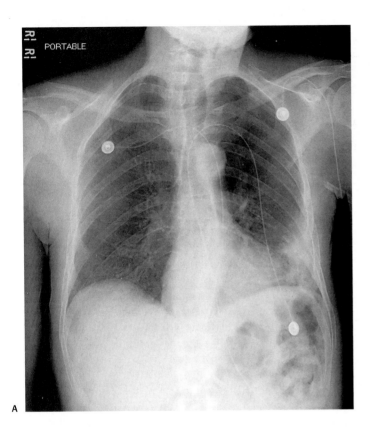

A

◼ Clinical Presentation

A 50-year-old man with cough who failed treatment with antibiotics.

Further Work-up

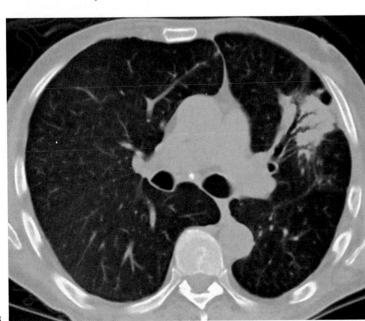

B

■ Imaging Findings

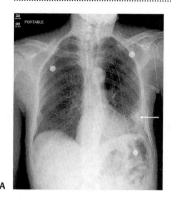

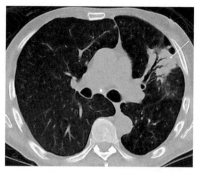

(A) Chest radiograph demonstrates peripheral left lung airspace opacity (*arrow*). **(B)** Computed tomography of the chest (lung windows) at the level of the carina (*arrow*) shows peripheral consolidation in the lingula.

■ Differential Diagnosis

- ***Cryptogenic organizing pneumonia (COP):*** Chronic subpleural consolidation that does not respond to antibiotic therapy makes COP a leading consideration.
- *Primary lung carcinoma:* Bronchoalveolar carcinoma can mimic COP. It may present with chronic consolidation but is usually not subpleural.
- *Lymphoma:* Pulmonary lymphoma is usually secondary to known disease. Lymphadenopathy would be expected.

■ Essential Facts

- COP presents with dyspnea, cough, and fever over a period of weeks.
- Many patients have a history of respiratory tract infection.
- Typically, there is a rapid response to corticosteroid treatment.
- Organizing pneumonia is associated with a variety of collagen vascular diseases, drug-induced lung disease, and infections.
- Intra-alveolar fibroblast proliferation results in patchy consolidation.
- Typically, there is peripheral or peribronchial consolidation with lower lobe predominance.

- There may be ground-glass or air-space opacity with air bronchograms.
- Linear interstitial abnormality or cavitary nodules are seen in atypical cases.
- Pleural effusion is uncommon.
- The "reversed halo" sign is central ground-glass opacity with a rim of consolidation. The finding is nonspecific but has been described in COP.

✓ Pearls & ✗ Pitfalls

- ✓ Lung opacities may spontaneously migrate or resolve.
- ✓ The term *organizing pneumonia* refers to the morphologic pattern, whereas the term *COP* refers to the associated idiopathic clinical syndrome.
- ✗ COP was formerly known as bronchiolitis obliterans organizing pneumonia, although this term has fallen out of favor to avoid confusion with unrelated small-airway diseases.
- ✗ Bronchoalveolar lavage or biopsy may be necessary to exclude malignancy, chronic eosinophilic pneumonia, or pneumonia.

Case 73

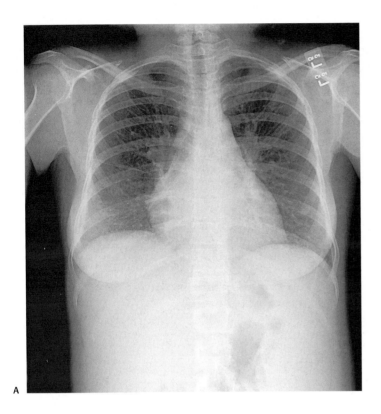

A

Clinical Presentation

A 45-year-old woman who has mixed connective tissue disease presenting with cough and fatigue.

Further Work-up

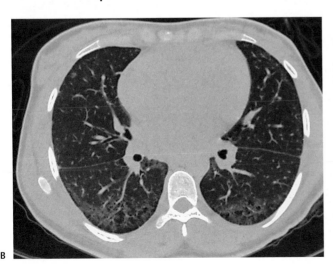

B

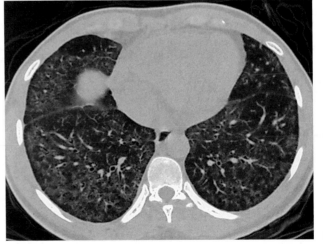

C

■ Imaging Findings

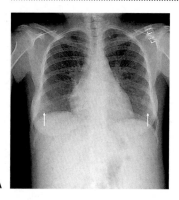 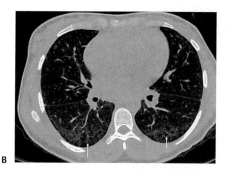 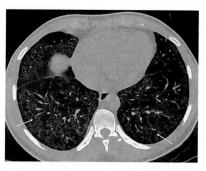

(A) Chest radiograph shows mild basilar opacity but is otherwise normal (*arrows*). **(B)** Computed tomography (CT) of the chest (lung windows) at the mid-thorax shows symmetric subpleural reticular opacities and micronodules (*arrows*). **(C)** CT of the chest (lung windows) at the lung bases shows more extensive reticular opacities, scattered areas of ground-glass opacity, and mild traction bronchiectasis (*arrows*).

■ Differential Diagnosis

- *Nonspecific interstitial pneumonia (NSIP):* NSIP is characterized by ground-glass opacity, reticular opacities, and micronodules. Radiologic evidence of NSIP is commonly found in patients with collagen vascular disease.
- *Hypersensitivity pneumonitis:* Chronic hypersensitivity pneumonitis can be difficult to distinguish from NSIP. Centrilobular nodules, mosaic attenuation, ground-glass opacity remote from areas of fibrosis, lack of significant honeycombing, and relative basal sparing are expected.
- *Desquamative interstitial pneumonia (DIP):* DIP is strongly associated with cigarette smoking. It is characterized by basal predominant ground-glass opacity. Honeycombing is uncommon, but well-defined, thin-walled cysts may develop.

■ Essential Facts

- The characteristic age is between 40 and 50 years.
- Symptoms are similar to those of idiopathic pulmonary fibrosis (IPF) but are usually milder.
- The NSIP pattern can be found in patients with collagen vascular diseases, hypersensitivity pneumonitis, and drug-induced lung disease.
- In contrast to patients with IPF, those with NSIP may respond to steroid treatment.

- The lower lobes are more frequently involved, although there is no distinct apicobasal gradient, as in usual interstitial pneumonia (UIP).
- A subpleural symmetric distribution is noted.
- There are ground-glass and reticular opacities.
- There are scattered nodules.
- Subpleural cysts can develop, resulting in what has been termed *microcystic honeycombing.*

✓ Pearls & ✗ Pitfalls

- ✓ Once the NSIP pattern is identified, secondary forms of NSIP, such as those due to collagen vascular disease, must be excluded clinically.
- ✓ Patients with fibrotic NSIP have a poorer prognosis than those with inflammatory histologic findings (cellular NSIP).
- ✗ Many patients with fibrosis and ground-glass opacity previously given a diagnosis of UIP with fibrosing alveolitis likely had NSIP rather than UIP.

Case 74

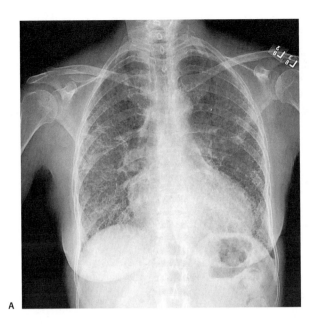

A

■ Clinical Presentation

A 62-year-old woman with progressive dyspnea.

Further Work-up

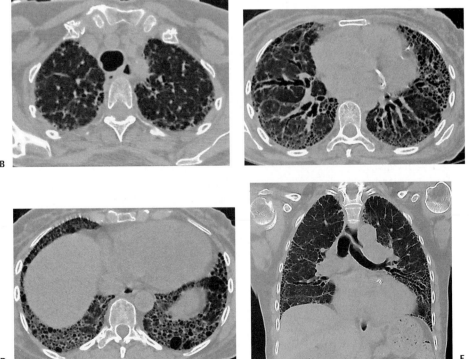

B C

D E

■ Imaging Findings

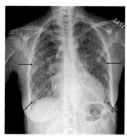 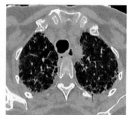 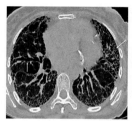 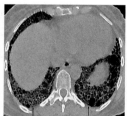 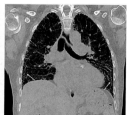

A–E

(A) Chest radiograph demonstrates symmetric base–predominant reticulation with volume loss (*arrows*). **(B)** Computed tomography (CT) of the chest (lung windows) through the lung apices demonstrates symmetric subpleural reticulation (*arrow*). **(C)** CT of the chest (lung windows) at the level of the aortic root shows more extensive traction bronchiectasis as well as honeycombing (*arrows*). There is no significant ground-glass component. **(D)** CT of the chest (lung windows) at the lung bases shows severe fibrosis and honeycombing (*arrows*). **(E)** CT of the chest (coronal) shows the subpleural and basilar distribution to advantage (*arrows*).

■ Differential Diagnosis

- ***Usual interstitial pneumonia (UIP):*** The basal peripheral predominance with extensive honeycombing makes UIP the best choice.
- *Hypersensitivity pneumonitis:* Chronic hypersensitivity pneumonitis can be difficult to distinguish from UIP. Centrilobular nodules, mosaic attenuation, ground-glass opacity remote from areas of fibrosis, lack of significant honeycombing, and relative basal sparing are expected.
- *Asbestosis:* Findings on high-resolution CT mimic findings of UIP. Curvilinear lines and subpleural bands are seen early on. Honeycombing is a common finding in advanced cases. Parietal pleural thickening is highly suggestive of asbestosis.

■ Essential Facts

- Idiopathic pulmonary fibrosis (IPF) is the clinical syndrome associated with the morphologic pattern of UIP.
- Patients are typically older than 50 years of age.
- UIP usually presents with progressive dyspnea and cough.
- The median survival time after diagnosis is less than 4 years.

- IPF does not respond to steroid treatment.
- IPF is the most common idiopathic interstitial pneumonia.
- In a patient with characteristic CT findings and clinical features, the diagnosis can be reliably made without biopsy.
- The chest radiograph shows decreased lung volumes and subpleural reticular opacities.
- On CT, macrocystic honeycombing, traction bronchiectasis, and architectural distortion are seen.
- The distribution is distinctly subpleural with an apicobasal gradient.

✓ Pearls & ✗ Pitfalls

- ✓ Nodularity, extensive ground-glass opacity, or consolidation suggests an alternative diagnosis.
- ✓ On serial examinations, areas of ground-glass opacity progress to fibrosis.
- ✗ Ground-glass opacity as a marker for alveolitis in inflammatory phase is no longer felt to be valid because UIP is primarily a fibrotic condition.
- ✗ Complications of IPF include infection, lung cancer, and accelerated deterioration.

Case 75

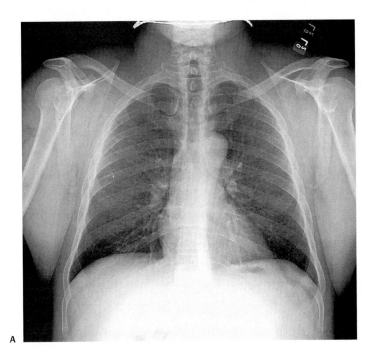

A

Clinical Presentation

A 55-year-old man with cough. He is a heavy smoker.

Further Work-up

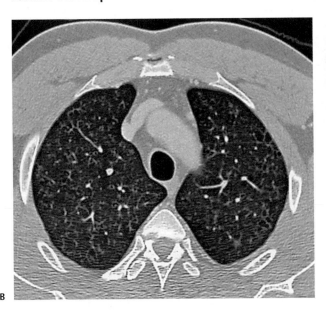

B

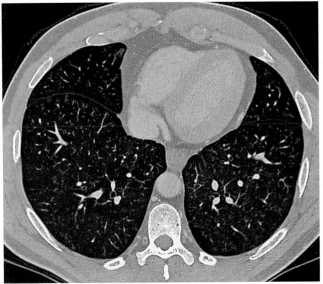

C

■ Imaging Findings

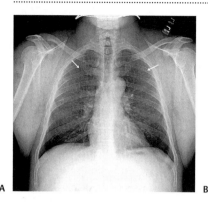 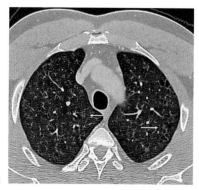 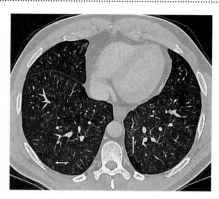

A   B   C

(A) Chest radiograph shows subtle, upper lobe–predominant, nodular interstitial abnormality (*arrows*). **(B)** Computed tomography (CT) of the chest (lung windows) at the lung apices demonstrates widespread bilateral centrilobular nodules on a background of centrilobular emphysema (*arrows*). **(C)** CT of the chest (lung windows) at the lung bases shows similar findings, but to a much lesser extent (*arrows*).

■ Differential Diagnosis

- *Respiratory bronchiolitis–interstitial lung disease (RB-ILD):* Upper lobe–predominant centrilobular nodules in a heavy smoker are suggestive of RB-ILD.
- *Hypersensitivity pneumonitis (HSP):* Although the imaging findings are similar, HSP is typically more widespread, with more obvious abnormalities. HSP is less likely in heavy smokers. Exposure to a specific antigen may be evident.
- *Pulmonary Langerhans cell histiocytosis:* This is also a smoking-related interstitial lung disease with upper lobe predominance. Characteristically, however, nodules and cysts are seen.

■ Essential Facts

- RB-ILD is a smoking-related interstitial lung disease.
- It is a symptomatic form of respiratory bronchiolitis.
- It shares features with desquamative interstitial pneumonia, which is part of the same continuum of smoking-related interstitial lung disease.

- RB-ILD typically affects men who are heavy smokers between the ages of 30 and 40 years.
- Symptoms regress with smoking cessation and, occasionally, steroid treatment.
- The chief abnormality is upper lobe–predominant centrilobular nodules.
- Ground-glass opacity and bronchial wall thickening also develop.
- There are usually no signs of fibrosis.
- Coexistent centrilobular emphysema is common.
- Air trapping is seen on expiratory-phase images.

✓ Pearls & ✗ Pitfalls

- ✓ Although the imaging appearance may mimic that of hypersensitivity pneumonitis, RB-ILD affects smokers, whereas most patients with HSP are nonsmokers.
- ✗ The imaging findings are indistinguishable from those of patients with asymptomatic respiratory bronchiolitis.
- ✗ The chest radiograph may be normal.

Case 76

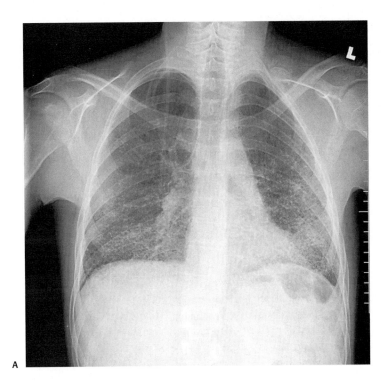

A

Clinical Presentation

A 40-year-old woman with dyspnea and recurrent aspiration.

Further Work-up

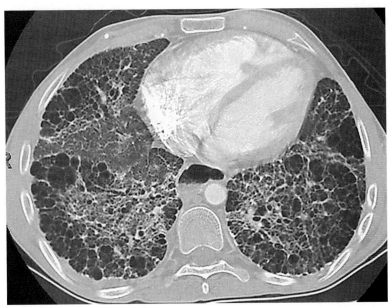

B

■ Imaging Findings

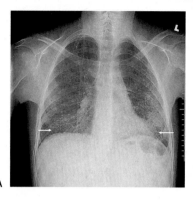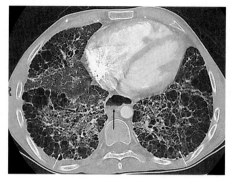

(A) Chest radiograph demonstrates lower lobe–predominant linear interstitial abnormality with small lung volumes (*arrows*). **(B)** Computed tomography of the chest (lung windows) at the lung bases shows extensive bilateral honeycombing and traction bronchiectasis (*white arrows*). The esophagus is severely dilated and contains an air-fluid level (*black arrow*).

■ Differential Diagnosis

- **Scleroderma:** Severe esophageal dilatation with lower lobe–predominant pulmonary fibrosis is highly suggestive of scleroderma.
- *Idiopathic pulmonary fibrosis:* This is not associated with esophageal dilatation. The distribution is classically subpleural.
- *Nonspecific interstitial pneumonia (NSIP):* Although there is significant overlap in the imaging findings, esophageal dilatation is not expected.

■ Essential Facts

- Scleroderma is characterized by the deposition of excessive extracellular matrix and vascular obliteration.
- The lung is the 4th most commonly involved organ, after the skin, arteries, and esophagus.
- A 3:1 female predominance is noted. Scleroderma typically presents by the age of 50 years.

- The course is progressive, with a high rate of mortality that is usually due to aspiration pneumonia.
- Pulmonary fibrosis is seen in up to 65% of patients.
- Fibrosis has a basilar predominance with a fine reticular pattern. This progresses to coarse reticulation with honeycombing.
- Ground-glass attenuation
- Poorly defined subpleural nodules
- Traction bronchiectasis
- Severely dilated esophagus
- Thin-walled subpleural cysts may be present.

✓ Pearls & ✗ Pitfalls

- ✓ Although the histologic patterns of usual interstitial pneumonia and NSIP can both be seen with scleroderma, that of NSIP is slightly more common.
- ✗ The prevalence of lung cancer is increased.

Case 77

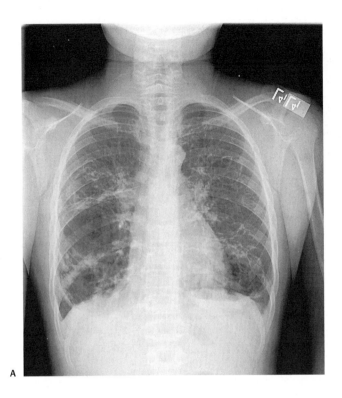

A

Clinical Presentation

A 10-year-old boy with wheezing and dyspnea.

Further Work-up

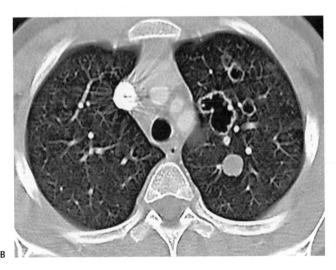

B

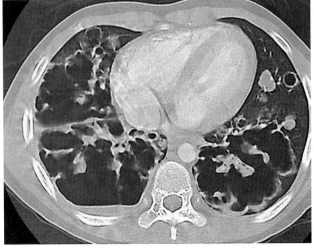

C

■ Imaging Findings

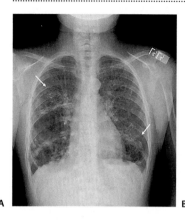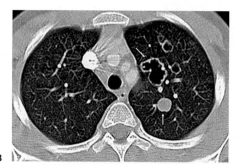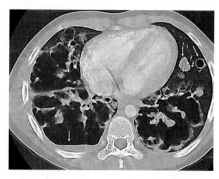

A   B   C

(A) Chest radiograph demonstrates multiple pulmonary nodules and extensive lower lobe–predominant cavities (*arrows*). **(B)** Computed tomography (CT) through the upper chest demonstrates a solid 2-cm nodule in the left upper lobe (*arrow*). Three irregularly shaped cavities are noted anterior to the nodule (*arrow*). The thickness of the walls is 3 to 4 mm. **(C)** CT through the lower chest demonstrates posteriorly predominant, large, thick–walled, irregular cavities with extensive parenchymal destruction. An air-fluid level is seen in the largest cavity on the right (*arrow*). Solid nodules (*medial arrow*) and a small, thin-walled cyst (*lateral arrow*) are seen in the anterior left lower lobe and lingula.

■ Differential Diagnosis

- **Pulmonary papillomatosis:** The patient's age, multiple nodules and cavities, and bilateral posterodorsal distribution favor papillomatosis.
- *Wegener granulomatosis:* This may also involve the trachea, but typically without frank nodularity. It can demonstrate widely distributed nodules of varying size that may cavitate. Patchy, shaggy air-space opacity and pulmonary hemorrhage can also be seen. These patients are typically older than those with papillomatosis.
- *Pulmonary Langerhans cell histiocytosis:* This also presents with nodules and cysts. However, there is a predilection for the upper lobes. The trachea is not involved. Pulmonary Langerhans cell histiocytosis typically occurs in adult smokers.

■ Essential Facts

- Pulmonary papillomatosis results from human papillomavirus (types 6 and 11) infection of the upper respiratory tract, most commonly acquired as a fetus passes through an infected birth canal.
- Adult sexual transmission can occur.
- Most cases remain limited to the trachea.
- Lung disease develops in 1% of cases, typically 10 years after laryngeal disease.

- Lung involvement may be secondary to the implantation of inhaled fragments from the larynx or multifocal viral infection.
- Laser therapy, antiviral medications, and surgical excision have been used to treat papillomatosis.
- The progression of disease can lead to respiratory failure.
- Multiple well-defined perihilar and posteriorly located nodules eventually cavitate.
- The lesions demonstrate extremely slow growth, measured in decades.
- Large intrabronchial lesions may cause obstructive atelectasis, pneumonia, or bronchiectasis.
- Nodular airway narrowing may be focal or diffuse.
- Solitary papillomas are rare and typically occur in adult male smokers.

✓ Pearls & ✗ Pitfalls

- ✓ Malignant degeneration to squamous cell carcinoma occurs in 10% of cases.
- ✓ An air-fluid level suggests superinfection.
- ✓ Any new or enlarging nodule should be evaluated further to exclude malignancy.
- ✗ Cavities may represent cavitary nodules, necrotic squamous cell carcinoma, or abscess secondary to obstructive pneumonitis.

Case 78

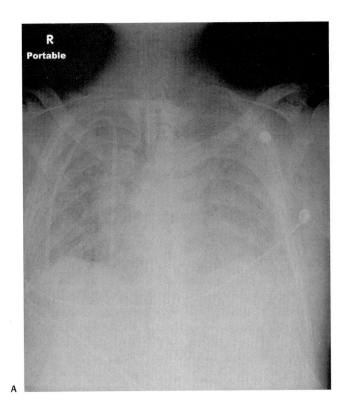

A

■ Clinical Presentation

A 50-year-old man with sepsis following bone marrow transplant.

Further Work-up

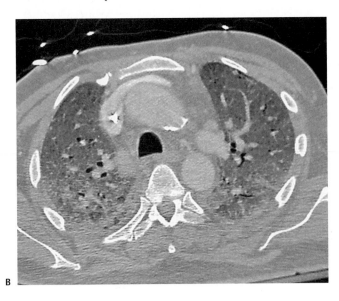

B

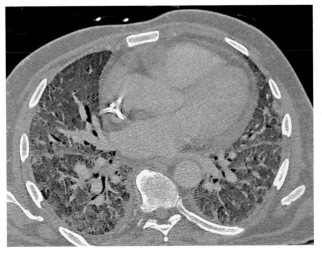

C

■ Imaging Findings

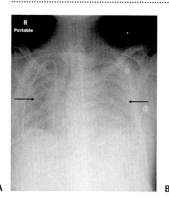
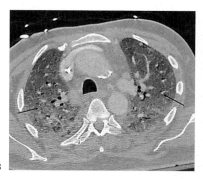
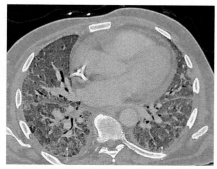

(A) Portable chest radiograph demonstrates an intubated patient with a right internal jugular central venous catheter (*arrows*). There is diffuse, bilateral pulmonary opacity without evidence of cardiomegaly or pleural effusion. **(B)** Contrast-enhanced computed tomography (CT; lung window) through the upper chest confirms widespread ground-glass opacity without pleural effusion or frank consolidation (*arrows*). **(C)** Contrast-enhanced CT (lung window) through the lower chest shows diffuse ground-glass opacity, mosaic attenuation, and pulmonary edema (*arrows*). Note the lack of pleural effusions and inhomogeneous distribution.

■ Differential Diagnosis

- ***Acute respiratory distress syndrome (ARDS):*** Diffuse, bilateral lung opacities without other evidence of congestive heart failure are suggestive of ARDS in this critically ill patient.
- *Hydrostatic pulmonary edema:* The imaging features of hydrostatic pulmonary edema and ARDS overlap, and without an adequate clinical history and knowledge of the arterial blood gas or pulmonary artery wedge pressure, differentiation can be difficult. However, hydrostatic pulmonary edema is classically associated with pleural effusions and cardiomegaly. The opacity found in cardiogenic edema is classically more centrally located.
- *Desquamative interstitial pneumonia:* This is a smoking-related idiopathic interstitial pneumonia characterized by diffuse lower lung zone–predominant ground-glass opacity. Although symptoms such as cough and dyspnea can be severe, respiratory distress requiring mechanical ventilation is not expected. The condition of most patients improves with smoking cessation and steroid treatment.

■ Essential Facts

- Diffuse pulmonary parenchymal injury is associated with noncardiogenic pulmonary edema.
- It results in severe respiratory distress and hypoxemic respiratory failure.
- ARDS is associated with a wide variety of clinical disorders that result in direct or indirect lung injury.
- Pneumonia, aspiration, trauma, fat and amniotic fluid embolism, inhalational injury, sepsis, drug overdose, and pancreatitis are among the best-documented causes.

- The diagnosis is made on clinical grounds: acute onset, bilateral lung opacity, pulmonary artery wedge pressure of 18 mm Hg or lower (or no clinical signs of congestive heart failure), and a Pao_2:Fio_2 ratio of 200 mm Hg or lower.
- The pathologic hallmark is diffuse alveolar damage.
- ARDS progresses through exudative, fibroproliferative, and fibrotic phases.
- The mortality rate approaches 60%.
- Nearly all patients have ground-glass opacity.
- Lung opacity is typically bilateral and dependent.
- Lung opacity evolves rapidly, with maximal severity in the first 3 days. It may progress to frank consolidation.
- Pneumothorax occurs in ~10% of cases and is not necessarily related to positive-pressure ventilation.
- In patients who survive, the ground-glass opacity and consolidation clear, although a reticular interstitial abnormality with architectural distortion and traction bronchiectasis may persist.

✓ Pearls & ✗ Pitfalls

- ✓ The most common risk factor for ARDS is sepsis.
- ✓ Pleural effusion is atypical and may suggest complicating pneumonia.
- ✓ The lack of cardiomegaly, septal lines, vascular redistribution, and peribronchial cuffing favor ARDS over cardiogenic edema.
- ✗ The term *acute interstitial pneumonia* is reserved for idiopathic cases of diffuse alveolar damage.
- ✗ The correlation between the imaging findings and the degree of hypoxemia is variable.

Case 79

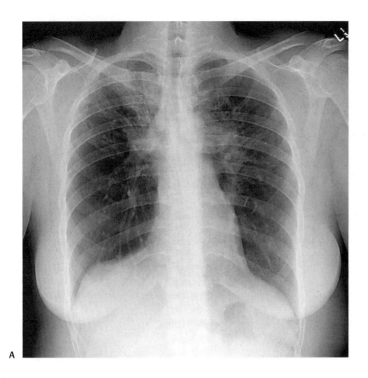

A

▨ Clinical Presentation

A 45-year-old woman with severe dyspnea.

Further Work-up

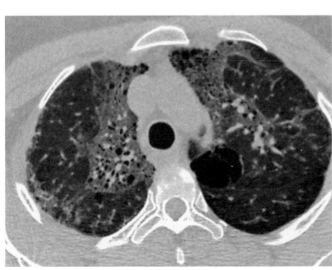

B

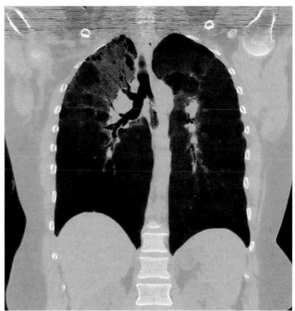

C

■ Imaging Findings

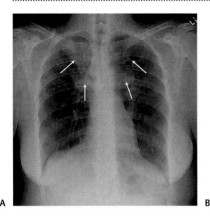
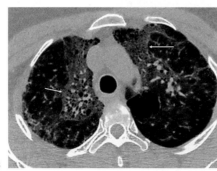
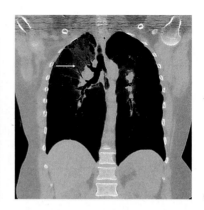

(A) Chest radiograph demonstrates an upper lobe–predominant interstitial abnormality with upper lobe retraction (*arrows*). There is mild paratracheal and hilar lymphadenopathy. **(B)** Computed tomography (CT) of the chest (lung windows) demonstrates severe upper lobe volume loss, traction bronchiectasis, and cyst formation (*arrows*). There is extensive subpleural nodularity. **(C)** CT of the chest (coronal minimum-intensity projection) demonstrates the striking upper lobe–predominant fibrosis to advantage (*arrow*).

■ Differential Diagnosis

- **Sarcoidosis:** The striking upper lobe predominance, small subpleural nodules, and lymphadenopathy make end-stage sarcoidosis the best choice.
- *Berylliosis:* This has a similar imaging appearance, although an appropriate occupational exposure (aerospace, electronics, and ceramics industries) should be elicited. Berylliosis is far less common than sarcoidosis.
- *Hypersensitivity pneumonitis (HP):* Chronic HP is typically more diffuse, although relative basal sparing is seen. The nodules are centrilobular, and more extensive ground-glass opacity is expected.

■ Essential Facts

- Sarcoidosis is an immunologically mediated multiple-organ granulomatous disease of unknown etiology.
- It is more common in females and African-Americans.
- It typically manifests in young and middle-aged adults.
- The clinical course and prognosis are highly variable.
- Fifty percent of patients are asymptomatic.
- Although almost any organ can be affected, intrathoracic involvement is seen in 90% of cases.
- Extrathoracic manifestations without intrathoracic disease occur in fewer than 10% of cases.
- Symmetric hilar and right paratracheal lymphadenopathy is the most common imaging finding. This is dubbed the "1, 2, 3" sign or "Garland triad." Nodes may calcify in an amorphous or eggshell pattern.
- High-resolution CT shows small perivascular nodules bilaterally, with irregular "beaded" thickening of the bronchovascular bundles and interlobular septa.
- Pulmonary involvement is typically upper lobe–predominant.
- End-stage disease results in architectural distortion, with upper lobe retraction, traction bronchiectasis, honeycombing, and cysts.

- Clinical staging can be based on the pattern of radiographic findings:
  - Stage 0: normal chest radiograph
  - Stage 1: lymphadenopathy only
  - Stage 2: lymphadenopathy and parenchymal disease
  - Stage 3: parenchymal disease only
  - Stage 4: pulmonary fibrosis
- Miliary nodules, bronchial wall thickening, and ground-glass opacity are less commonly seen.
- "Alveolar sarcoidosis" demonstrates large peripheral opacities with air bronchograms.

■ Other Imaging Findings

- Activity on gallium 67 scan results in the "lambda" sign, with paratracheal and hilar uptake, and the "panda" sign, with lacrimal and parotid uptake.
- Fluorodeoxyglucose uptake is variable in intensity and pattern.

✓ Pearls & ✗ Pitfalls

- ✓ Beaded interlobular septal thickening can also occur in lymphangitic carcinomatosis, but in contrast to that seen in sarcoidosis, it is not associated with lobular architectural distortion and is unlikely to have a perihilar distribution.
- ✓ The combination of erythema nodosum, arthralgia, and intrathoracic lymphadenopathy is called Löfgren syndrome.
- ✗ Silicosis may have a similar imaging appearance, although an appropriate occupational exposure (mining, stone, and glass industries) should be elicited.
- ✗ The major complications of sarcoidosis are fibrosis, cor pulmonale, and mycetoma formation.
- ✗ In addition to the overlap in imaging findings with lymphadenopathy, a lymphoproliferative disorder is more than five times more likely to develop in patients with sarcoidosis.

Case 80

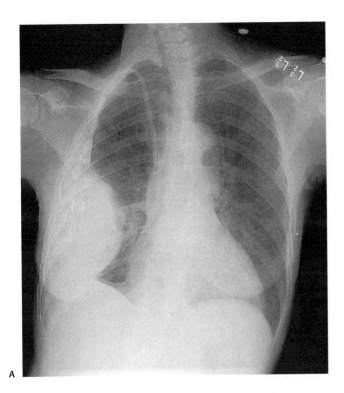

A

■ Clinical Presentation

A 40-year-old woman with fever and an elevated white cell count.

Further Work-up

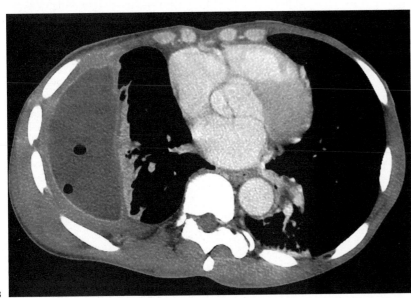

B

■ Imaging Findings

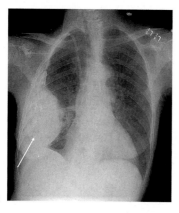
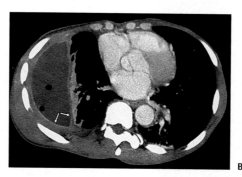

A   B

(A) Posteroanterior chest radiograph demonstrates a large pleura-based mass on the right (*arrow*). A hemodialysis catheter is in the expected location. **(B)** Contrast-enhanced computed tomography (CT; soft-tissue windows) demonstrates a loculate pleural effusion containing air. The pleura is thickened and hyperdense (*arrows*).

■ Differential Diagnosis

- **Empyema:** Pleural thickening and enhancement surrounding a pleural effusion are highly suggestive of an empyema.
- *Mesothelioma:* This typically results in a rind thicker than 1 cm. Extension into the fissures or along mediastinal pleural surfaces is common. Pleural effusion is common, although infectious signs and symptoms are usually absent. Mesothelioma may be associated with calcified pleural plaques indicative of asbestos exposure.
- *Pulmonary abscess:* This occurs within the lung parenchyma rather than in the pleural space.

■ Essential Facts

- The visceral pleura covers the lungs and forms the interlobar fissures. The parietal pleura covers the diaphragm, mediastinum, and inner surface of the thoracic cage. There is only a thin layer of fluid within the pleural space, and the pleural surfaces are typically not identified on radiography or CT.
- Exudative pleural effusions have an elevated specific gravity and high levels of protein and lactate dehydrogenase. They typically have infectious, inflammatory, or neoplastic causes.
- Transudative pleural effusions are typically due to congestive heart failure, renal failure, cirrhosis, nephrotic syndrome, or hypoproteinemia.
- Thoracic empyema is defined as purulent content in the pleural cavity.
- It typically results from the transformation of a parapneumonic pleural effusion and undergoes three stages. In the exudative stage, the fluid is sterile, and the glucose level and pH are normal. In the fibrinopurulent stages, the glucose level and pH decrease as white cells and bacteria accumulate in the fluid. In the chronic organizing stage, the

exudate is thick and purulent, and a fibrin peel develops. The pleural peel can organize as early as at 7 days.
- The development of air pockets within the pleural fluid may indicate a bronchopleural fistula.
- The "split pleura" sign refers to thickened visceral and parietal pleural layers separated by fluid. Although not specific for empyema, it does indicate that an exudative pleural effusion is present.

■ Other Imaging Findings

- CT is highly accurate at differentiating an empyema from a lung abscess. An empyema is typically oblong, with a smooth inner margin that displaces surrounding lung. An abscess is usually a thick-walled spherical cavity that is completely surrounded by lung and forms an acute angle with the pleura.
- Enhancement of the pleura is usually seen.
- Ultrasound may help visualize internal septa and debris.
- If the initial response to tube drainage is not successful, fibrinolytics can be infused to facilitate evacuation. Video-assisted thoracoscopic surgery or open drainage may be required in complex cases.

✓ Pearls & ✗ Pitfalls

- ✓ There is usually associated thickening and increased attenuation of the extrapleural fat.
- ✓ Tuberculous empyema can result in thick calcification and rib thickening.
- ✗ Empyema necessitans is spontaneous decompression of an empyema through the chest wall. It is most common in tuberculous and fungal empyema.
- ✗ If the underlying lung is noncompliant, it may not re-expand following drainage, resulting in a "trapped lung."

Case 81

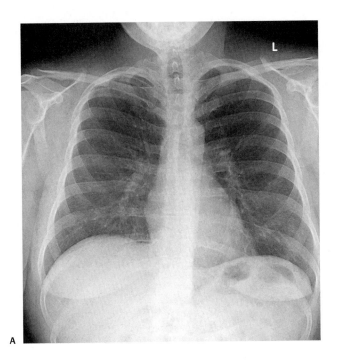

A

Clinical Presentation

A 32-year-old woman with progressive dyspnea.

Further Work-up

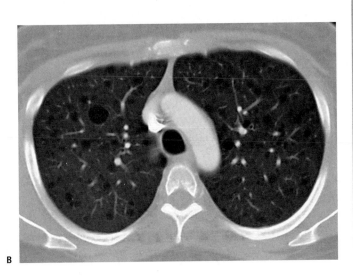

B

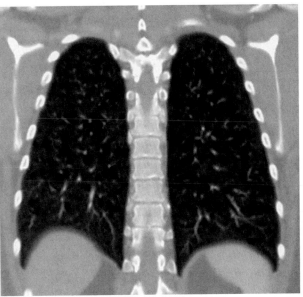

C

■ **Imaging Findings**

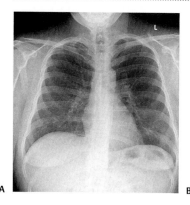
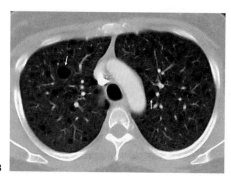
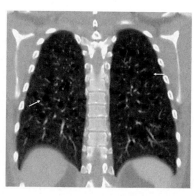

A   B   C

(A) Chest radiograph is normal. **(B)** Computed tomography (CT) of the chest (axial, lung windows) shows diffusely scattered thin-walled cysts (*arrows*). The intervening lung is normal. **(C)** CT of the chest (coronal, lung windows) demonstrates that the cysts are diffusely scattered and affect the lung bases (*arrows*).

■ **Differential Diagnosis**

- *Lymphangioleiomyomatosis (LAM):* The diffuse distribution of thin-walled cysts in a woman of childbearing age makes LAM the best choice.
- *Tuberous sclerosis (TS):* Lung involvement with TS has an appearance identical to that of LAM. Patients with TS would be expected to manifest multiple other findings, such as seizures, mental retardation, facial angiofibromas, cortical tubers, and subependymal nodules. It is hypothesized that LAM and TS are two forms of the same disease.
- *Pulmonary Langerhans cell histiocytosis (PLCH):* Cysts in PLCH have variable thickness. There are usually associated nodules with varying degrees of cavitation. The costophrenic angles are spared. PLCH occurs in smokers.

■ **Essential Facts**

- LAM occurs exclusively in females, typically of childbearing age.
- There is a proliferation of smooth muscle in the pulmonary lymphatics, vessels, and airways.
- LAM commonly presents with dyspnea on exertion or pneumothorax.
- The course is variable but typically slowly progressive.
- Cysts (usually round and thin-walled) are uniformly distributed and seen in all cases.
- The parenchyma between the cysts is normal.

- Reticulation may be seen on chest radiographs, and this is due to the summation of numerous cysts and interstitial edema.
- Recurrent pneumothorax and chylothorax are commonly encountered.
- Lung volumes are large.
- Abdominal findings are present in 70% of cases and consist of renal angiomyolipomas, retroperitoneal cystic masses (lymphangioleiomyomas), lymphadenopathy, and chylous ascites.

✓ **Pearls & ✗ Pitfalls**

✓ The size of the cysts may decrease on expiratory-phase scans.
✓ Chylous effusion may be suggested on CT when the fluid has a low (< 0 Hounsfield units) attenuation.
✓ The thoracic duct may be markedly enlarged.
✗ Hemorrhage is seen in ~10% of cases.
✗ Following transplant, recurrent LAM can develop in the donor lung in rare cases.

Case 82

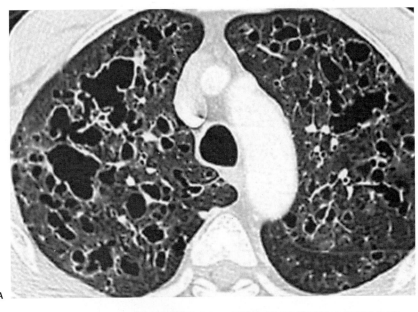

A

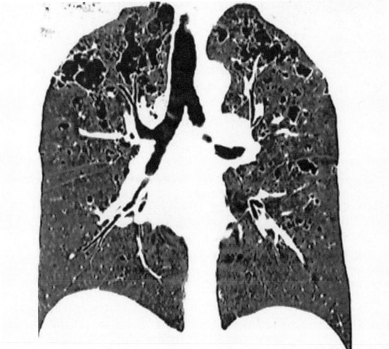

B

■ Clinical Presentation

A 32-year-old man who is a smoker with fatigue and chronic cough.

■ Imaging Findings

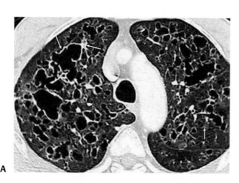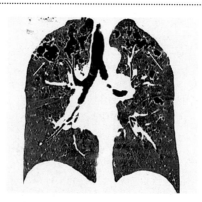

A　　　　　　　　　　　　　　　　　　　　　　　　　　　　　　　B

(A) Computed tomography (CT) of the chest (axial, lung windows) shows bilateral irregularly shaped cysts and scattered nodules (*arrows*). **(B)** CT of the chest (coronal re-formation) demonstrates upper lobe predominance. The lung bases are not affected (*arrows*).

■ Differential Diagnosis

- ***Pulmonary Langerhans cell histiocytosis (PLCH):*** Irregularly shaped, upper lobe–predominant cysts with variable wall thickness and scattered indistinct nodules in a young male smoker make PLCH the best choice.
- *Lymphangioleiomyomatosis (LAM):* LAM is characterized by diffusely distributed thin-walled cysts. It occurs exclusively in females.
- *Laryngotracheal papillomatosis:* This presents with cysts and nodules, although usually in a dependent distribution. Laryngeal and tracheal nodules may be seen.

■ Essential Facts

- PLCH has been referred to as histiocytosis X, eosinophilic granuloma, Letterer-Siwe disease, and Hand-Schüller-Christian syndrome, among many other names.
- A peribronchiolar proliferation of Langerhans cells (from the monocyte-macrophage line) results in granulomatous infiltration. It is believed that in certain individuals, an allergic reaction to cigarette smoke stimulates cytokine production and Langerhans cell activation.
- On microscopy, Birbeck granules with their characteristic "tennis racquet" appearance are seen.
- PLCH typically affects young adult smokers.
- Treatment centers on smoking cessation. Corticosteroids are occasionally administered. The clinical course is unpredictable.
- Symmetric upper lobe–predominant nodules are characteristic. The costophrenic sulci are spared.

- Lung volumes are normal to increased.
- Recurrent pneumothorax is not uncommon.
- A progression of imaging abnormalities may be seen on CT: nodules, cavitary nodules, thick-walled cysts, thin-walled cysts, and finally confluent cysts.
- The cysts assume a wide variety of shapes.
- Nodules are usually smaller than 1 cm. They are rarely seen in isolation.
- Lymphadenopathy and consolidation are rarely seen.
- As in LAM and other cystic lung disease, the cysts may decrease in size on expiratory-phase images as a consequence of communication with the airways.
- Rib involvement (lytic expansile lesions with beveled edges) may be seen.

✓ Pearls & ✗ Pitfalls

- ✓ A predominantly nodular pattern is seen in early phases, whereas a cystic pattern is most evident in later phases.
- ✓ As opposed to the nodules in sarcoidosis, silicosis, and lymphangitic carcinomatosis, those in PLCH are usually centrilobular.
- ✗ It may be difficult to distinguish emphysema from cysts on radiographs.
- ✗ Pneumatoceles from *Pneumocystis* pneumonia can appear identical to cysts found in PLCH.
- ✗ PLCH may recur in transplanted lungs if smoking is continued.

Case 83

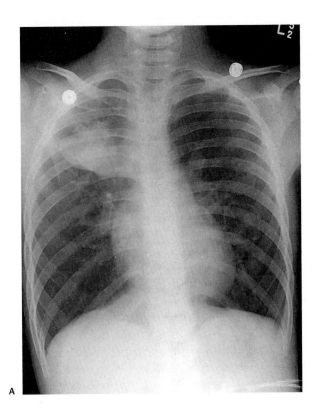

A

■ Clinical Presentation

A 15-year-old boy with worsening dyspnea.

Further Work-up

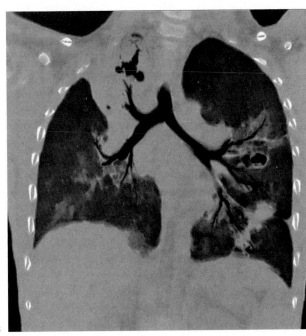

B

■ Imaging Findings

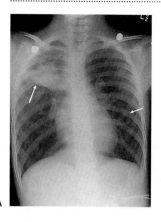

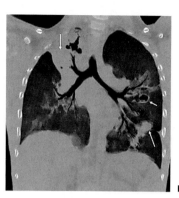

A

B

(A) Chest radiograph demonstrates multiple pulmonary nodules and a cavitary nodule in the left lung (*arrows*). (B) Computed tomography of the chest (coronal re-formation) shows the right upper lobe consolidation to advantage. The cavitary nodule in the left upper lobe has a thin but irregular wall. Solid nodules are also seen in the left lower lobe (*arrows*).

■ Differential Diagnosis

- ***Pulmonary papillomatosis:*** The patient's age and the multiple nodules and cavities favor papillomatosis.
- *Pulmonary Langerhans cell histiocytosis (PLCH):* PLCH can also present with nodules and cysts; typically, the lung volumes are large, and there is a predilection for upper lobe involvement. There is a strong association with cigarette smoking.
- *Lymphangioleiomyomatosis (LAM):* LAM is characterized by diffusely distributed, thin-walled cysts. It occurs exclusively in females.

■ Essential Facts

- Pulmonary papillomatosis results from human papillomavirus (types 6 and 11) infection of the upper respiratory tract, acquired most commonly as a fetus passes through an infected birth canal.
- Adult sexual transmission can occur.
- Most cases remain limited to the trachea.
- Lung disease develops in 1% of cases, typically 10 years after laryngeal disease.
- Lung involvement may be secondary to the implantation of inhaled fragments from the larynx or multifocal viral infection.

- Laser therapy, antiviral medications, and surgical excision have been used to treat papillomatosis.
- The progression of disease can lead to respiratory failure.
- Multiple well-defined perihilar and posteriorly located nodules eventually cavitate.
- The lesions demonstrate extremely slow growth, measured in decades.
- Large intrabronchial lesions may cause obstructive atelectasis, pneumonia, or bronchiectasis.
- Nodular airway narrowing may be focal or diffuse.
- Solitary papillomas are rare and typically occur in adult male smokers.

✓ Pearls & ✗ Pitfalls

- ✓ Malignant degeneration to squamous cell carcinoma occurs in 10% of cases.
- ✓ An air-fluid level suggests superinfection.
- ✓ Any new or enlarging nodule should be evaluated further to exclude malignancy.
- ✗ Cavities may represent cavitary nodules, necrotic squamous cell carcinoma, or abscess secondary to obstructive pneumonitis.

Case 84

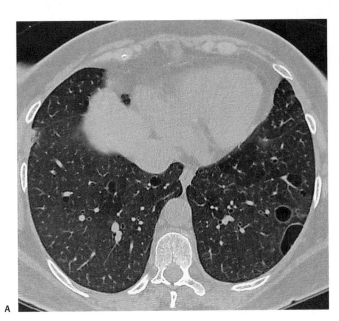

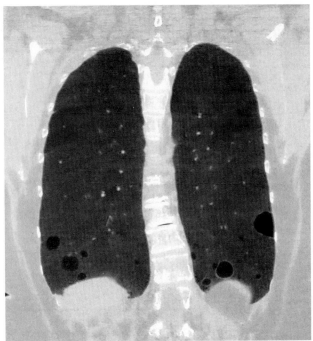

A

B

▪ Clinical Presentation

A 55-year-old woman with Sjögren disease and chronic dyspnea.

■ Imaging Findings

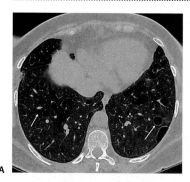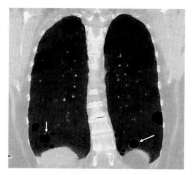

A   B

(A) Computed tomography (CT) of the chest (lung windows) at the lung bases shows randomly distributed thin-walled cysts (*arrows*). There are scattered small centrilobular nodules, minimal ground-glass opacity, and mild bronchial wall thickening. **(B)** CT of the chest (coronal minimum-intensity projection) shows the distribution of the thin-walled cysts to advantage (*arrows*).

■ Differential Diagnosis

• *Lymphoid interstitial pneumonia (LIP):* Scattered ground-glass opacity and random thin-walled cysts in a patient with Sjögren syndrome are highly suggestive of LIP.
• *Nonspecific interstitial pneumonia (NSIP):* Although ground-glass opacities and a micronodular pattern may be seen, thin-walled cysts are not typically present in NSIP.
• *Hypersensitivity pneumonitis (HP):* Although ground-glass attenuation and small centrilobular nodules are seen in HP, the presence of thin-walled cysts argues against this diagnosis. An appropriate exposure to a specific antigen may be evident, although not always.

■ Essential Facts

• LIP is a rare benign lymphoproliferative disorder.
• Most commonly associated with Sjögren syndrome, acquired immunodeficiency syndrome (AIDS), or Castleman disease
• More common in women
• Slowly progressive cough and dyspnea

• Variable response to corticosteroids
• Very rarely evolves into B-cell lymphoma
• Lower lobe–predominant centrilobular nodular opacities
• Bilateral ground-glass opacities
• Randomly distributed thin-walled cysts
• Mild lymphadenopathy is seen in the majority of cases.
• Thickened bronchovascular bundles and interlobular septal thickening are seen on high-resolution CT.
• Fibrosis and honeycombing are rare.
• Except for the cysts, the radiologic abnormalities may resolve with successful treatment.

✓ Pearls & ✗ Pitfalls

✓ Nodules are more common in patients infected with human immunodeficiency virus.
✓ Cysts are thought to develop as a consequence of the obstruction of bronchioles by lymphocytic infiltrate.
✗ It can be difficult to differentiate LIP from *Pneumocystis* pneumonia in patients with AIDS. Although both result in ground-glass opacities and cysts, the presence of interlobular septal thickening and lymphadenopathy favor LIP.
✗ LIP is an AIDS-defining illness in children, but not adults.

Case 85

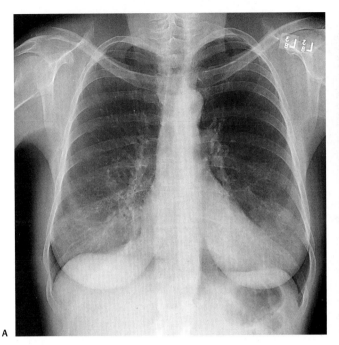

A

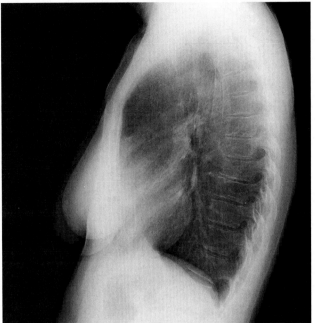

B

▪ Clinical Presentation

A 67-year-old woman with chronic cough.

Further Work-up

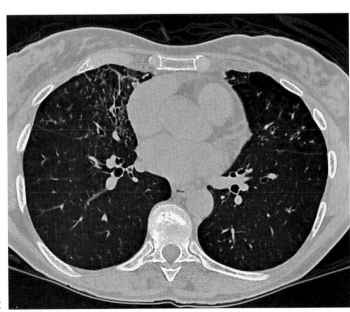

C

■ Imaging Findings

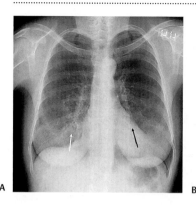
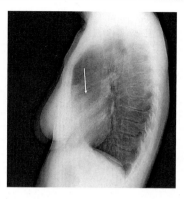
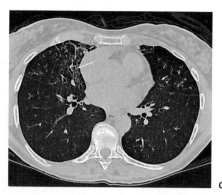

A   B   C

(A) Posteroanterior chest radiograph demonstrates mild interstitial opacity in the medial lower lung fields (*arrows*). **(B)** Lateral chest radiograph localizes bronchiectasis and interstitial opacity to the right middle lobe and lingula (*arrow*). **(C)** Computed tomography (CT) of the chest (lung windows) demonstrates centrilobular nodules, tree-in-bud opacity, bronchial wall thickening, and bronchiectasis in the right middle lobe (*arrow*) and lingula.

■ Differential Diagnosis

- ***Nontuberculous mycobacteria (NTMB) infection:*** Centrilobular nodules, tree-in-bud opacity, bronchial wall thickening, and bronchiectasis are compatible with bronchiolitis. In this case, infectious bronchiolitis is expected, and with the patient's demographics and symptoms, an NTMB infection with an agent such as *Mycobacterium avium-intracellulare* (MAI) is the most likely diagnosis.
- *Histoplasmosis:* Although common, histoplasmosis usually results in randomly distributed nodules that often calcify. Lymphadenopathy is also commonly seen.
- *Sarcoidosis:* This classically manifests as upper lobe–predominant perilymphatic nodules with lymphadenopathy.

■ Essential Facts

- NTMB typically infect the lungs, lymph nodes, and skin.
- They usually cause chronic low-grade infections.
- The most common NTMB infections are due to MAI, *Mycobacterium kansasii*, and *Mycobacterium xenopi*.
- NTMB are ubiquitous, but human-to-human transmission is rare.
- NTMB infection is divided into five groups:
  - Classic infection with upper lobe–predominant consolidation, nodularity, and cavitation
  - Nonclassic infection with centrilobular nodules and bronchiectasis
  - Solitary or clustered granulomas in asymptomatic patients
  - Pneumonia in an immunosuppressed host
  - Infection in a patient with achalasia

- Classic infection typically affects elderly men with chronic obstructive pulmonary disease.
- Nonclassic infection is frequently due to MAI and affects elderly women without underlying lung disease. This has been termed the "Lady Windermere" syndrome.
- In patients with acquired immunodeficiency syndrome, lymphadenopathy is the most common finding. Infection usually does not occur until the CD4-cell count is below $70/mm^3$.
- In classic infection, cavitation is common and frequently seen in the upper lobes.
- Nonclassic infection is characterized by imaging findings of bronchiolitis: bronchial wall thickening, bronchiectasis, centrilobular nodules, tree-in-bud opacity, and air trapping. Nodules are usually smaller than 1 cm.

✓ Pearls & ✗ Pitfalls

- ✓ Nonclassic infection is usually most severe in the lingula and right middle lobe.
- ✓ Patients with achalasia are predisposed to *Mycobacterium fortuitum-chelonae* infection, which results in dependent confluent bilateral opacity.
- ✗ The tree-in-bud or "toy jack" pattern on high-resolution CT is compatible with bronchiolitis but is a nonspecific finding with a broad differential diagnosis.
- ✗ Post-primary tuberculosis can have an identical imaging appearance, although bronchiectasis is usually less extensive. The purified protein derivative skin test result may be positive in patients with NTMB infection.

Case 86

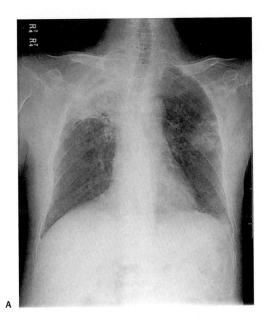

A

■ Clinical Presentation

A 45-year-old man with fever and hemoptysis.

Further Work-up

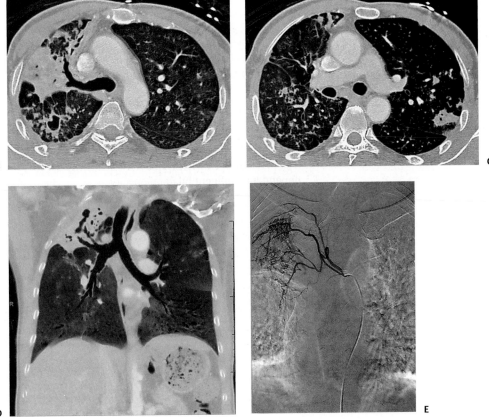

B

C

D

E

■ Imaging Findings

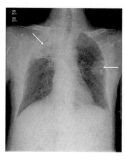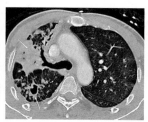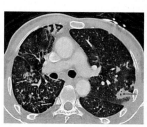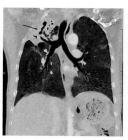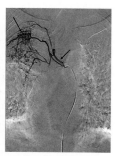

A–E

(A) Posteroanterior chest radiograph demonstrates dense right upper lobe consolidation with a suggestion of cavitation (*arrows*). **(B)** Contrast-enhanced computed tomography (CT) of the chest (lung windows) at the level of the aortic arch confirms the right upper lobe consolidation (*arrow*). There is a thick-walled, cavitary mass in the superior segment of the right lower lobe. It is surrounded by multiple centrilobular nodules and tree-in-bud opacity. **(C)** Contrast-enhanced CT of the chest (lung windows) at the level of the pulmonary artery shows multiple nodules on the left, the largest of which appears cavitary (*black arrow*). On the right, there are diffusely scattered centrilobular nodules and areas of bronchial wall thickening (*white arrows*). **(D)** Minimum-intensity-projection CT of the chest (coronal re-formation) shows the right upper lobe consolidation and cavitation to advantage (*arrow*). **(E)** Right bronchial angiogram shows severely hypertrophic bronchial arteries with an irregular parenchymal blush (*arrows*).

■ Differential Diagnosis

- **Postprimary tuberculosis (TB):** Widespread upper lobe consolidation and cavitation in association with findings of bronchiolitis, such as centrilobular nodules and bronchial wall thickening, make TB the diagnosis of exclusion.
- *Bronchogenic carcinoma:* Primary lung cancer can mimic TB in cases with cavitation, adenopathy, and chronic lung opacity. In this case, the bilateral nature of the findings makes primary lung cancer unlikely. However, endobronchial spread of carcinoma can result in tree-in-bud opacity and centrilobular nodules.
- *Atypical mycobacterial pneumonia:* Atypical mycobacterial pneumonia can appear identical to infection with *Mycobacterium tuberculosis*. Given the necessity of isolating patients with TB, it is the diagnosis of exclusion.

■ Essential Facts

- TB is usually confined to the respiratory system.
- Primary TB is seen in patients not previously exposed to the organism. It typically manifests as middle or lower lobe consolidation.
- Postprimary TB refers to both reinfection and reactivation TB.
- Postprimary TB manifests as consolidation, usually in the apical and posterior segments of the upper lobes. Cavitation is seen in 50% of cases.
- Lymphadenopathy is rare in postprimary TB.

- As little as 300 mL per day is considered massive hemoptysis.
- The source of bleeding is the bronchial arteries in 90% of cases.
- Aspergillomas can develop in cavities.
- The bronchial arteries arise at or near the level of the left main bronchus in 94% of cases.
- Particles are the preferred embolic agent.

✓ Pearls & ✗ Pitfalls

- ✓ Cavitation is the hallmark of postprimary disease.
- ✓ Rasmussen aneurysm is a pulmonary artery aneurysm due to adjacent cavitary TB.
- ✓ Coils are typically not used as embolic agents because they prevent future attempts at embolization when symptoms recur.
- ✗ Inadvertent embolization of the greater anterior medullary artery (artery of Adamkiewicz) can result in paralysis. It usually arises near the T9 to T12 spinal level, somewhat lower than the bronchial arteries.
- ✗ The pulmonary artery and nonbronchial systemic arteries can be the source of bleeding in a minority of cases.
- ✗ Particles that are too small can pass through shunts and result in pulmonary artery and systemic embolization.
- ✗ Broncholithiasis, pericardial involvement, fibrosing mediastinitis, fibrothorax, and chest wall involvement are additional sequelae of TB.

Case 87

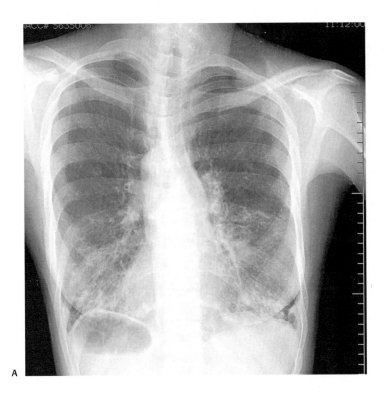

A

■ Clinical Presentation

A 37-year-old woman with chronic cough and infertility.

Further Work-up

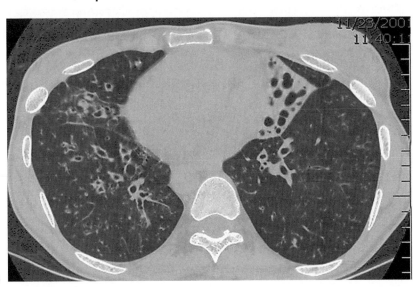

B

■ Imaging Findings

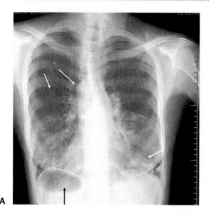
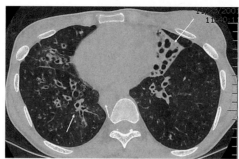

(A) Posteroanterior chest radiograph demonstrates bilateral lower lobe–predominant bronchiectasis and bronchial wall thickening. There is a basally predominant nodular interstitial pattern. The aortic arch, cardiac apex, and stomach bubble are right-sided (*arrows*). **(B)** Noncontrast computed tomography (CT) of the chest (lung windows) through the lung bases confirms widespread bronchiectasis and bronchial wall thickening. There are multiple centrilobular nodules and areas of tree-in-bud opacity. There is consolidation in the "left middle lobe" in this patient with situs inversus (*arrows*).

■ Differential Diagnosis

- **Primary ciliary dyskinesia:** Lower lobe–predominant bronchiectasis is seen in primary ciliary dyskinesia. Fifty percent of these patients have situs inversus.
- *Cystic fibrosis:* Bronchiectasis is usually upper lobe–predominant. Infertility is also present. Cystic fibrosis is typically more severe and progressive, and patients present earlier in life. There is no association with situs inversus.
- *Williams-Campbell syndrome:* This is a congenital disorder of defective cartilage in the 4th to 6th bronchial generations, presenting either diffusely or in one focal area of lung. The lung distal to the bronchiectasis may be emphysematous. There are no extrathoracic manifestations, and situs inversus is not expected.

■ Essential Facts

- Primary ciliary dyskinesia encompasses a spectrum of ciliary abnormalities, including ciliary akinesia, dyskinesia, and aplasia.
- Typical clinical manifestations include chronic cough, rhinitis, and sinusitis. Cilia dysfunction results in impaired mucociliary clearance.
- The inheritance pattern is autosomal-recessive. Most men are infertile because of immotile spermatozoa.
- Patients can be screened by measuring exhaled nasal nitric oxide (minimal or absent); however, a definitive diagnosis requires electron microscopy to confirm specific defects. Genetic testing is available for specific mutations.
- Situs inversus occurs in approximately half of patients (body asymmetry is randomized) with immotile cilia syndrome and is not an essential part of the disorder.

- Moderate hyperinflation, bronchial thickening, and bronchiectasis are the most common imaging findings.
- Small centrilobular nodules are often seen on high-resolution CT (HRCT).
- Bronchiectasis is classified into three categories: cylindric, varicose, and cystic.
- The "signet ring" sign refers to visualization of a dilated bronchus adjacent to the pulmonary artery on cross-section.
- Nasal polyps and aplasia of the frontal sinuses are features.
- Primary ciliary dyskinesia is associated with congenital cardiac abnormalities such as transposition of the great vessels. Pyloric stenosis and epispadias are other associations.

✓ Pearls & ✗ Pitfalls

- ✓ Kartagener syndrome is a subtype of primary ciliary dyskinesia in which situs inversus, sinusitis, and bronchiectasis occur together.
- ✓ Lack of bronchial tapering or visualization of bronchi within 1 cm of the pleura may be early findings of bronchiectasis on HRCT.
- ✗ Bronchiectasis may not manifest until adulthood.
- ✗ Primary ciliary dyskinesia often results in recurrent pneumonia and scarring. Mycetoma formation and hemorrhage may ensue.

Case 88

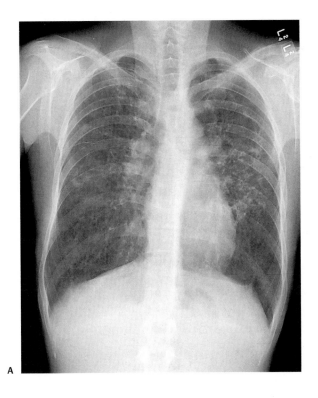

A

■ Clinical Presentation

A 21-year-old man with chronic cough.

Further Work-up

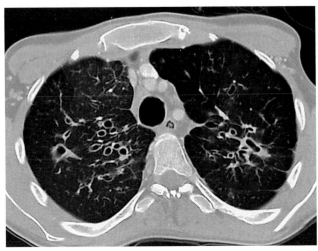

B

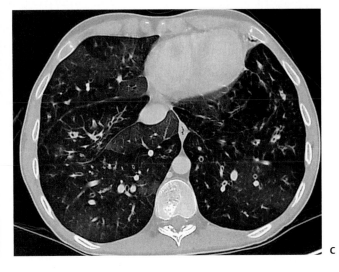

C

■ Imaging Findings

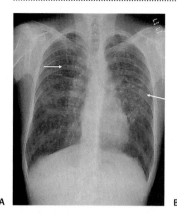
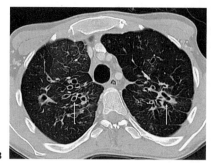
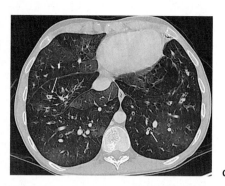

(A) Posteroanterior chest radiograph demonstrates bilateral upper lobe–predominant bronchial wall thickening and bronchiectasis (*arrows*). The lung volumes are relatively large. **(B)** Contrast-enhanced computed tomography (CT) through the upper lobes confirms upper lobe bronchial wall thickening and bronchiectasis (*arrows*). **(C)** Contrast-enhanced CT through the lower lobes demonstrates mosaic attenuation. Bronchial wall thickening and bronchiectasis, although present, are not as severe as in the upper lobes (*arrows*).

■ Differential Diagnosis

- **Cystic fibrosis (CF):** Upper lobe–predominant bronchial wall thickening and bronchiectasis in a patient of this age are highly suggestive of CF.
- *Allergic bronchopulmonary aspergillosis (ABPA):* ABPA manifests as upper lobe–predominant central bronchiectasis in patients with asthma. ABPA develops in approximately 10% of patients with CF.
- *Kartagener syndrome:* Ciliary dysmotility disorders result in diffuse bronchiectasis. In Kartagener syndrome, situs inversus and sinusitis are also present.

■ Essential Facts

- CF is an autosomal-recessive disease seen primarily in Caucasians. It is due to a gene defect that affects chloride transport across cell membranes, resulting in thick mucus.
- Most cases are detected by early childhood with a sweat chloride test.

- Bronchial wall thickening, bronchiectasis, and mucous plugging are commonly seen.
- Lung volumes are generally increased.
- Pleural effusions are rare.
- Mosaic attenuation is due to small-airways disease. Air trapping can be seen on expiratory-phase CT.
- Bronchiolar obstruction also results in centrilobular nodules and tree-in-bud opacity.
- There is fatty or cystic replacement of the pancreas.
- The central pulmonary arteries are enlarged.

✓ Pearls & ✗ Pitfalls

- ✓ The lower lobes are less severely affected because of the more efficient clearance of secretions.
- ✓ The right upper lobe is usually the most severely affected.
- ✓ Meconium ileus at birth is highly suggestive of CF.
- ✗ Recurrent pneumonia is often due to *Pseudomonas*.
- ✗ Lung abscess and hemoptysis requiring bronchial artery embolization are additional complications.

Case 89

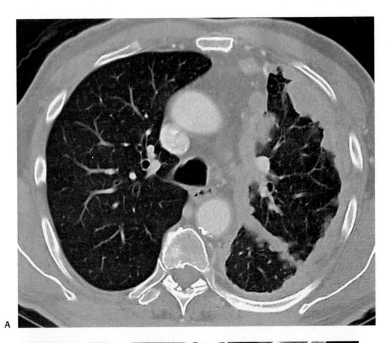

A

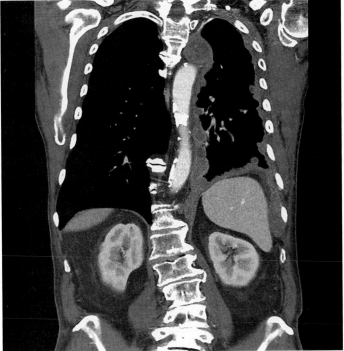

B

◼ Clinical Presentation

A 66-year-old man with progressive dyspnea. He is a mechanic.

■ Imaging Findings

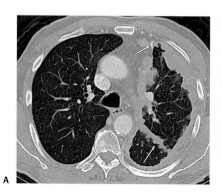
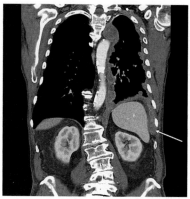

(A) Contrast-enhanced computed tomography (CT; lung windows) demonstrates circumferential left-sided pleural thickening. Extensive nodularity is seen involving the left minor fissure (*arrows*). Note the very small focus of calcification anteriorly. The right hemithorax is normal. (B) Noncontrast CT (coronal re-formation, soft-tissue windows) shows extension deep into the costophrenic angle (*arrow*). Note the volume loss in the left hemithorax.

■ Differential Diagnosis

- **Mesothelioma:** Unilateral pleural thickening with volume loss and extension into the fissure is highly suggestive of mesothelioma, especially in a patient with a significant history of asbestos exposure.
- *Metastatic adenocarcinoma:* Adenocarcinoma metastatic to the pleura cannot be reliably differentiated from mesothelioma based on imaging alone. Pleural effusion is slightly less common with metastases.
- *Empyema:* Although pleural effusion and thickening are also seen in empyema, the circumferential distribution, nodularity, thickening of more than 1 cm, and involvement of the mediastinal pleura are findings that favor malignancy.

■ Essential Facts

- Mesothelioma is the most common primary neoplasm of pleura. It occurs in up to 10% of persons exposed to asbestos (risk factor of 30 compared with the general population).
- Although all types of asbestos have been linked to mesothelioma, crocidolite (an amphibole fiber) is the most carcinogenic because of its aspect ratio (length to diameter) and durability in tissue. The incidence of mesothelioma is highest in those with the longest and most severe exposure. There is no association with cigarette smoking.
- High-risk occupations include insulation work, asbestos manufacturing, heating trades, shipyard work, and automotive brake lining manufacture and repair.
- The latency period is 30 to 40 years.
- Mesothelioma is histologically divided into epithelioid, sarcomatous, and biphasic variants. The parietal pleura is involved to a much greater degree.
- Unilateral pleural and fissural thickening associated with pleural effusion are the hallmark imaging findings.
- Circumferential encasement involving all pleural surfaces is a late manifestation.
- Chest wall invasion manifests radiographically as periosteal reaction or rib erosion/destruction but is identified in only 20% of cases. CT adds sensitivity, and obliteration of

the extrapleural fat plane and invasion of the intercostal muscles may also be demonstrated.
- Lung parenchymal and hilar/mediastinal nodal metastases are evidence of advanced disease.
- Transdiaphragmatic extension is suggested by encasement of the hemidiaphragm and the loss of clear fat planes within the abdominal organs.

■ Other Imaging Findings

- Magnetic resonance imaging can help detect invasion of the diaphragm or chest wall. Lesions are usually minimally hyperintense to muscle on T1-weighted and moderately hyperintense on T2-weighted images.
- Fluorodeoxyglucose positron emission tomography may aid the preoperative evaluation because of its high sensitivity in detecting extrathoracic metastases. It can also provide information about metabolically active areas and therefore determine the most appropriate area for biopsy.
- Extrapleural pneumonectomy is performed in selected cases but is associated with significant morbidity and mortality. Results of radiation therapy and chemotherapy have been disappointing. The median survival of patients with mesothelioma is 10 months.

✓ Pearls & ✗ Pitfalls

- ✓ "Frozen hemithorax" describes the lack of contralateral mediastinal shift in association with massive pleural effusion due to encasement of the lung and fissures by neoplasm.
- ✓ Despite asbestos exposure, calcified pleural plaques are seen in only 20% of cases.
- ✗ The term *benign mesothelioma* has been used to describe a localized fibrous tumor of the pleura. Its use is discouraged because this lesion is a separate entity and histologically benign. There is no association with asbestos exposure.
- ✗ Pleural fluid cytology and fine-needle aspiration are not sufficient for diagnosis. Video-assisted thoracoscopic surgery can result in chest wall seeding in 50% of patients. This can be prevented with local postoperative radiation therapy.

Case 90

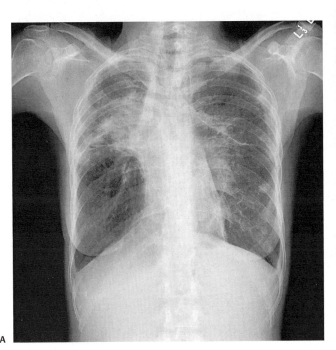

A

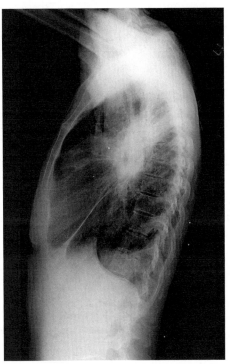

B

Clinical Presentation

A 50-year-old woman with severe dyspnea and an elevated angiotensin-converting enzyme level.

Further Work-up

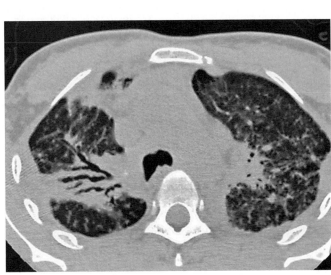

C

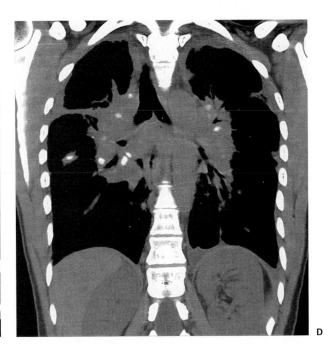

D

■ **Imaging Findings**

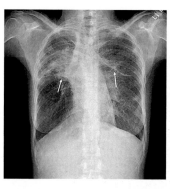 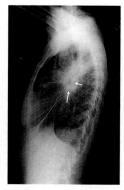 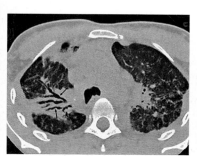 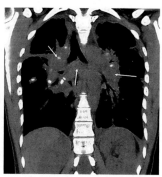

A–D

(A) Posteroanterior chest radiograph demonstrates hilar and paratracheal lymphadenopathy with upper lobe retraction (*arrows*). **(B)** Lateral chest radiograph shows the lymphadenopathy to advantage (*arrows*). **(C)** Computed tomography (CT) of the chest (lung windows) shows areas of consolidation with traction bronchiectasis on the right (*right arrows*). In the left upper lobe, there are widespread perilymphatic nodules and thickening of the bronchovascular bundles (*left arrow*). **(D)** CT of the chest (coronal, soft-tissue window) best shows the extensive calcified lymphadenopathy (*arrows*).

■ **Differential Diagnosis**

- *Sarcoidosis:* Calcified hilar and mediastinal lymphadenopathy and upper lobe–predominant perilymphatic nodules are suggestive of sarcoidosis.
- *Idiopathic pulmonary fibrosis:* Although associated with severe reticulation and traction bronchiectasis, the hallmark finding is honeycombing. The abnormalities are characteristically most severe at the lung bases. Calcified lymph nodes are not expected.
- *Pulmonary Langerhans cell histiocytosis (LCH):* Although upper lobe–predominant lung disease is seen with LCH, this typically demonstrates large lung volumes with cysts and nodules. Lymphadenopathy is uncommon. It is almost exclusively seen in smokers.

■ **Essential Facts**

- Sarcoidosis is an immunologically mediated multiple-organ granulomatous disease of unknown etiology.
- It is more common in females and African Americans.
- It typically manifests in young and middle-aged adults.
- The clinical course and prognosis are highly variable.
- Fifty percent of patients are asymptomatic.
- Angiotensin-converting enzyme is a product of macrophages and an indicator of granulomatous activity. It is elevated in 70% of patients.
- Symmetric hilar and right paratracheal lymphadenopathy is the most common imaging finding. This is dubbed the "1, 2, 3" sign or "Garland triad."
- Nodal calcification is related to duration of disease. Nodes may calcify in an amorphous or eggshell pattern.
- High-resolution CT shows small perivascular nodules bilaterally, with irregular "beaded" thickening of the bronchovascular bundles and interlobular septa.
- Pulmonary involvement is typically upper lobe–predominant.

- End-stage disease results in architectural distortion, with upper lobe retraction, traction bronchiectasis, honeycombing, and cysts.
- Clinical staging can be based on the pattern of radiographic findings:
  - Stage 0: normal chest radiograph
  - Stage 1: lymphadenopathy only
  - Stage 2: lymphadenopathy and parenchymal disease
  - Stage 3: parenchymal disease only
  - Stage 4: pulmonary fibrosis
- Miliary nodules, bronchial wall thickening, and ground-glass opacity are less commonly seen.
- "Alveolar sarcoidosis" demonstrates large peripheral opacities with air bronchograms.

■ **Other Imaging Findings**

- Activity on gallium 67 scan results in the "lambda" sign, with paratracheal and hilar uptake, and the "panda" sign, with lacrimal and parotid uptake.
- Fluorodeoxyglucose uptake is variable in intensity and pattern.

✓ **Pearls & ✗ Pitfalls**

- ✓ Beaded interlobular septal thickening can also occur in lymphangitic carcinomatosis, but in contrast to that seen in sarcoidosis, it is not associated with lobular architectural distortion and is unlikely to have a perihilar distribution.
- ✓ The combination of erythema nodosum, arthralgia, and intrathoracic lymphadenopathy is called Löfgren syndrome.
- ✗ The major complications of sarcoidosis are fibrosis, cor pulmonale, and mycetoma formation.
- ✗ In addition to the overlap in imaging findings with lymphadenopathy, a lymphoproliferative disorder is more than five times more likely to develop in patients with sarcoidosis.

Case 91

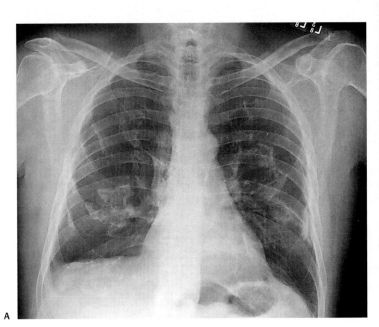

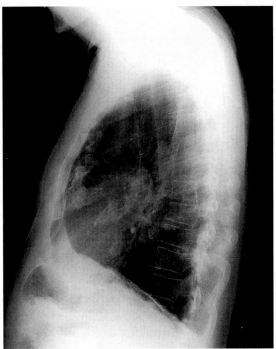

A

B

■ Clinical Presentation

An 80-year-old man with cough and dyspnea.

Further Work-up

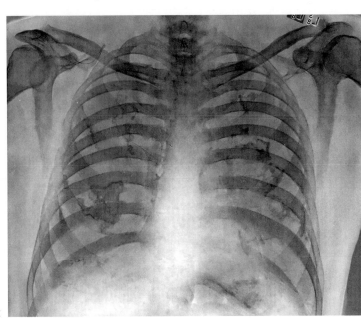

C

■ Imaging Findings

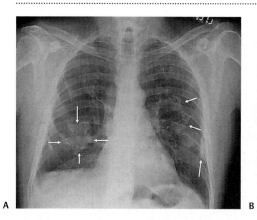
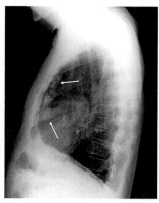
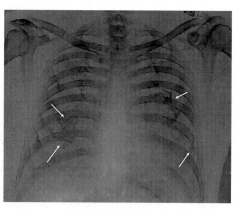

A   B   C

(A) Posteroanterior (PA) chest radiograph demonstrates irregularly shaped areas of calcification bilaterally (*arrows*). The diaphragmatic surfaces are also involved. **(B)** Lateral chest radiograph shows that the calcification is distributed along the pleural surfaces (*arrows*). **(C)** Energy-subtracted views from the PA radiograph show the calcification to advantage (*arrows*).

■ Differential Diagnosis

- *Calcified pleural plaques secondary to asbestos exposure:* Bilateral, thin, calcified pleural plaques in this distribution are compatible with calcified pleural plaques, which are highly suggestive of asbestos exposure.
- *Pleural calcification secondary to previous hemothorax:* This is often associated with imaging evidence of previous trauma or surgery. It is usually unilateral.
- *Mesothelioma:* This typically manifests as unilateral pleural thickening of less than 1 cm and is associated with a pleural effusion. Circumferential involvement and ipsilateral hemithoracic volume loss may be present.

■ Essential Facts

- Asbestos is a naturally occurring, fire-resistant silicate used in insulation, brake pads, floor tiles, and electric wiring. The biohazard arises from inhalation of the fibers during mining and processing. Amphibole fibers are more hazardous because of their durability and geometry.
- Asbestos exposure can result in pleural effusion, pleural plaques, diffuse pleural thickening, asbestosis, malignant mesothelioma, and bronchogenic carcinoma.
- Benign pleural effusion is the earliest pleura-based finding. It is usually self-limited.

- Pleural plaques are discrete areas of fibrosis involving the parietal pleura and the most common manifestation of asbestos exposure. They typically occur 20 to 30 years after exposure. Patients are usually asymptomatic, even if the plaques are widespread. The plaques are not associated with malignant mesothelioma.
- Pleural plaques are typically bilateral and multifocal. They preferentially involve the posterolateral parietal pleura, the dome of the diaphragm, and the mediastinal pleura. The apices and costophrenic angles are usually spared.
- Approximately 15% of plaques are calcified. The amount of calcification can increase with time.
- When a plaque is viewed in profile, a linear band of attenuation is seen. However, when seen en face, the plaque assumes an irregular, "holly leaf" configuration.

✓ Pearls & ✗ Pitfalls

- ✓ The term *hairy plaque* describes a visceral pleural plaque with short interstitial lines radiating into the adjacent lung parenchyma.
- ✗ The term *asbestosis* refers to lung fibrosis caused by asbestos and may not be associated with pleural fibrosis.

Case 92

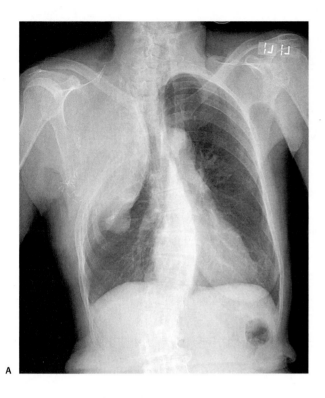

A

Clinical Presentation

An 80-year-old woman with dyspnea and a positive purified protein derivative test result.

Further Work-up

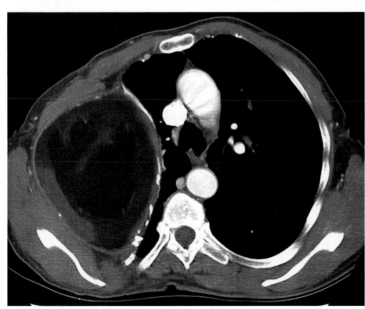

B

■ Imaging Findings

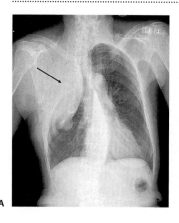
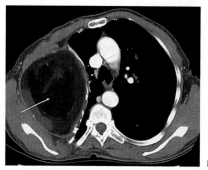

(A) Chest radiograph demonstrates severe deformity of the right chest wall and ribs, multiple surgical clips, right-sided volume loss, and a large mass in the right upper hemithorax (*arrow*). **(B)** Contrast-enhanced computed tomography (soft-tissue windows) shows a heterogeneous but predominant fat-density mass in the right hemithorax (*arrow*).

■ Differential Diagnosis

- ***Plombage:*** The patient previously underwent thoracoplasty. The large fat-density mass is compatible with wax plombage.
- *Locally advanced lung cancer:* Superior sulcus tumors can present with extensive rib destruction. Fat within the lesion is not compatible with lung cancer.
- *Mesothelioma:* This presents with pleural effusion and circumferential pleural thickening. Hemithoracic volume loss is present. Mesothelioma can result in chest wall destruction. A large fat-density mass is not compatible with mesothelioma.

■ Essential Facts

- Before the advent of effective antimycobacterial therapy, cavitary tuberculosis was sometimes treated with plombage.
- This therapy was curative in up to 75% of cases.
- In thoracoplasty, rib resection is performed to approximate the chest wall to the underlying lung, effectively collapsing the lung and obliterating the pleural space.

- In plombage, the extrapleural space is created and enlarged with foreign bodies. Typically, paraffin wax or polymethyl methacrylate spheres are used.
- Plombage has the advantage of preserving lung function and resulting in less/no physical deformity.
- Complications of extrapleural plombage include acute oil embolism, local infection, plombage migration, and mediastinal compression.
- Hemorrhage through vascular erosion and pleurocutaneous fistula can also result.
- Oleothorax has lipid density (< 0 Hounsfield units).
- Chronic hypoxia can result in pulmonary hypertension.

✓ Pearls & ✗ Pitfalls

- ✓ With the spread of multidrug-resistant tuberculosis, collapse therapy is again considered a treatment option.
- ✗ A bronchopleural fistula can result in the aspiration of oil and lipoid pneumonia.
- ✗ Secondary malignant tumors can result.

Case 93

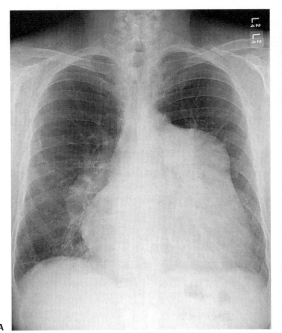
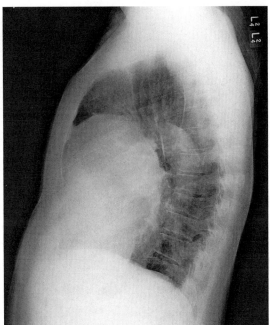

A

B

Clinical Presentation

A 52-year-old man with dyspnea on exertion.

Further Work-up

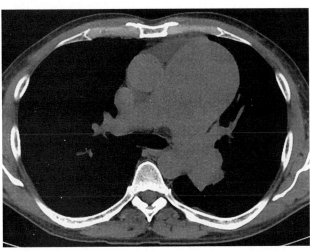
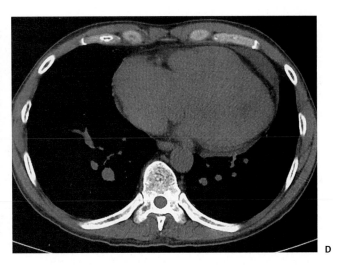

C

D

■ Imaging Findings

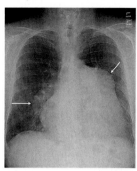
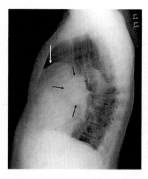
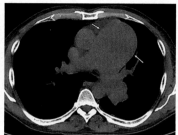
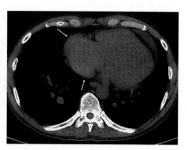

A–D

(A) Posteroanterior chest radiograph demonstrates cardiomegaly and massive central pulmonary artery enlargement (*arrows*). There is no evidence of pulmonary edema or pleural effusion. **(B)** Lateral chest radiograph confirms dilated right and left main pulmonary arteries (*black arrows*). Note the filling of the retrosternal clear space, a sign of right ventricular enlargement (*white arrow*). **(C)** Noncontrast computed tomography (CT) of the chest (soft-tissue windows) at the level of the main pulmonary artery confirms the significantly enlarged main pulmonary artery (*arrows*). Note the size discordance in comparison with the aorta. **(D)** Noncontrast CT of the chest (soft-tissue windows) through the heart shows the right-sided cardiac enlargement to advantage (*arrows*).

■ Differential Diagnosis

- **Pulmonary hypertension:** The abnormality of the cardio-mediastinal silhouette is due to massive central pulmonary artery enlargement. Right-sided cardiomegaly is a consequence of long-standing pulmonary hypertension.
- *Sarcoidosis:* Severe lymphadenopathy can initially be mistaken for pulmonary artery enlargement on frontal radiograph. However, the normal thickness of the right paratracheal stripe and lack of subcarinal adenopathy make adenopathy unlikely in this case. The lateral radiograph and CT confirm that it is, indeed, the pulmonary arteries that are enlarged. End-stage sarcoidosis can result in pulmonary hypertension.
- *Pulmonary valve stenosis:* Enlargement is usually isolated to the main and left pulmonary arteries.

■ Essential Facts

- Pulmonary hypertension is defined as mean pulmonary artery pressure higher than 25 mm Hg at rest (> 30 mm Hg during exercise). Normal mean pulmonary artery pressure is 10 mm Hg.
- Pulmonary hypertension is a result of vascular abnormalities within the arterial (precapillary) or venous (postcapillary) pulmonary circulation.
- Precapillary pulmonary hypertension is usually caused by long-standing left-to-right cardiac shunts, chronic thromboembolic disease or widespread pulmonary embolism, and collagen vascular disease.
- Postcapillary pulmonary hypertension is usually secondary to abnormalities of the left side of the heart, such as mitral stenosis or left ventricular failure. Pulmonary veno-occlusive disease is a rare idiopathic cause of postcapillary pulmonary hypertension. Because of transmission of the elevated pulmonary venous pressure across the capillary bed, pulmonary arterial hypertension may coexist.

- The imaging features of precapillary pulmonary hypertension include dilatation of the central pulmonary arteries, pruned vascularity, mosaic perfusion, and atherosclerosis of the pulmonary arteries.
- In mosaic perfusion, the caliber of vessels in hypoattenuated lung is decreased.
- The imaging features of postcapillary pulmonary hypertension include prominent interlobular septa, subpleural edema, and pleural effusions.
- On CT, the transverse diameter of the main pulmonary artery exceeds 29 mm.
- Dilatation of the right atrium and ventricle, thickening of the anterior right ventricular wall, and flattening of the interventricular septum are CT manifestations of cor pulmonale.
- The right interlobar artery is enlarged (> 16 mm in men and > 14 mm in women).

✓ Pearls & ✗ Pitfalls

- ✓ Primary pulmonary hypertension is a rare disorder occurring primarily in middle-aged women. There is a likely a genetic component, and the disorder has been associated with human immunodeficiency virus infection, the use of appetite suppressants, the use of cocaine, and portal hypertension.
- ✓ Scleroderma is the most common collagen vascular disease to cause pulmonary hypertension.
- ✓ Although not common in the United States, schistosomiasis is endemic in the Middle East, Africa, and Caribbean and can result in cirrhosis, portal hypertension, and pulmonary hypertension. Pulmonary hypertension is the result of parasite embolism and subsequent vascular inflammation.
- ✗ If vasodilators are administered to patients with pulmonary veno-occlusive disease, life-threatening pulmonary edema can result.

Case 94

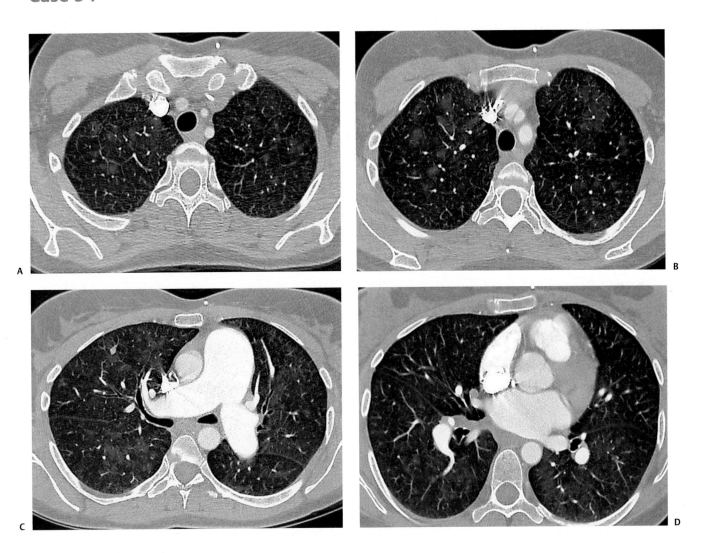

A

B

C

D

■ Clinical Presentation

A 45-year-old woman with dyspnea on exertion and normal pulmonary capillary wedge pressure.

■ Imaging Findings

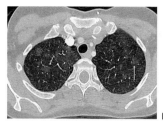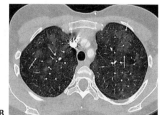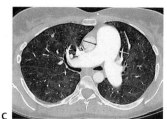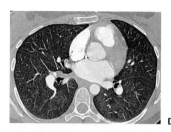

A   B   C   D

(A) Contrast-enhanced computed tomography (CT) of the chest (lung windows) through the apices demonstrates bilateral smooth interlobular septal thickening and scattered centrilobular ground-glass opacities (*arrows*). **(B)** Contrast-enhanced CT of the chest (lung windows) through the upper lobes shows more significant bilateral ground-glass opacity (*arrows*). **(C)** Contrast-enhanced CT of the chest (lung windows) at the level of the main pulmonary artery demonstrates a significantly enlarged main pulmonary artery (*black arrow*). Note the size discordance in comparison with the aorta. Interlobular septal thickening and ground-glass opacity are also seen at this level (*white arrow*). **(D)** Contrast-enhanced CT of the chest (lung windows) through the heart also shows very mild lymphadenopathy (*arrows*). The left atrium and visualized pulmonary veins are normal.

■ Differential Diagnosis

- **Pulmonary veno-occlusive disease (PVOD):** The combination of pulmonary hypertension, normal wedge pressure, smooth interlobular septal thickening, and centrilobular ground-glass nodules make PVOD the best choice.
- *Pulmonary edema:* Smooth interlobular septal thickening and ground-glass opacity are commonly seen in cardiogenic pulmonary edema. The wedge pressure would be expected to be elevated. Although long-standing left heart failure can result in pulmonary hypertension, in this case, the findings suggest isolated pulmonary hypertension.
- *Erdheim-Chester disease:* This is a non–Langerhans cell histiocytosis of unknown origin characterized by osteosclerotic bone lesions, perirenal encasement, and pleural or diffuse septal interstitial lung disease. Septal thickening can cause it to mimic veno-occlusive disease. However, the central pulmonary arteries would not be expected to be enlarged.

■ Essential Facts

- PVOD is a rare idiopathic cause of pulmonary hypertension characterized by intimal fibrosis that narrows and occludes the pulmonary veins.
- It typically affects children and young adults but has been reported in a wide range of ages.
- It is associated with viral infection, chemotherapy, autoimmune diseases, and bone marrow transplant.
- Enlarged pulmonary arteries are almost always present.
- Smooth interlobular septal thickening is seen.
- Centrilobular ground-glass nodular opacities are diffusely distributed.

■ Other Imaging Findings

- On angiography, the central pulmonary arteries are enlarged and the distal arterial branches are mildly narrowed. No filling defects should be seen.
- Pericardial and pleural effusions may be present.
- Mild lymphadenopathy has also been reported.

✓ Pearls & ✗ Pitfalls

- ✓ It is debated whether PVOD and pulmonary capillary hemangiomatosis (PCH) are distinct diseases. There is significant overlap in the imaging findings of PVOD and those of PCH. Septal lines are more numerous in PVOD, and ground-glass nodules are better circumscribed in PCH.
- ✓ Hemoptysis and hemorrhagic pleural effusions have been reported in PCH, but not in PVOD.
- ✓ The low wedge pressure helps differentiate PVOC and PCH from other causes of post-capillary pulmonary hypertension, such as left atrial myxoma, mitral stenosis, and pulmonary vein stenosis.
- ✗ PVOD and PCH are clinically indistinguishable from primary pulmonary hypertension. High-resolution CT is recommended before therapy is initiated because if vasodilators are administered to patients with PVOD, life-threatening pulmonary edema can result.
- ✗ Ventilation-perfusion scans have a varied appearance and can mimic "high-probability" scans, misdiagnosing chronic thromboembolic disease.

Case 95

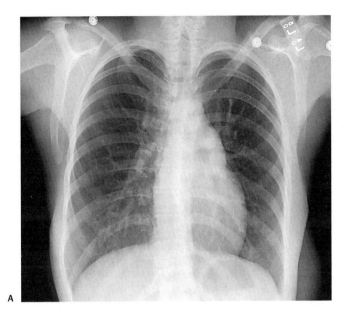

A

■ Clinical Presentation

A 22-year-old woman with decreased exercise tolerance.

Further Work-up

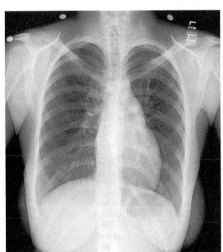

B

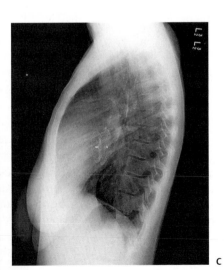

C

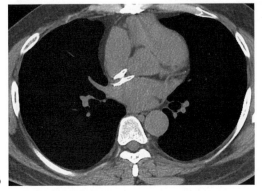

D

■ Imaging Findings

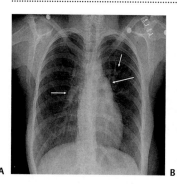
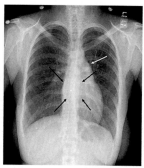
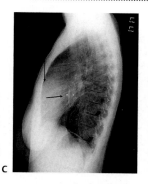
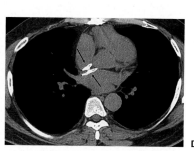

(A) Posteroanterior (PA) chest radiograph demonstrates enlargement of the main and central pulmonary arteries (*arrows*). There is increased pulmonary vascularity. **(B)** Following an intervention, the PA chest radiograph demonstrates normal pulmonary vascularity. The pulmonary artery, however, remains enlarged. An Amplatzer septal occluder device has been placed (*arrows*). **(C)** On the lateral chest radiograph, the occluder device is more easily visualized. Filling of the retrosternal clear space is due to right ventricular hypertrophy (*arrows*). **(D)** Noncontrast computed tomography of the chest obtained in a different patient with similar pathology shows the septal occluder to advantage. Note that the left atrial disk is larger than the right atrial disk (*arrows*).

■ Differential Diagnosis

- **Atrial septal defect (ASD):** The chest radiographic findings are compatible with shunt vascularity and pulmonary hypertension, making ASD the best choice.
- *Lymphadenopathy:* Lymphadenopathy in the anteroposterior window or prevascular space may create an abnormality in the mediastinal silhouette that can be mistaken for pulmonary artery enlargement. Shunt vascularity would not be expected.
- *Cor pulmonale:* Cor pulmonale refers to pulmonary hypertension and right ventricular dysfunction (usually hypertrophy) as the result of a respiratory disorder. There is no evidence of pulmonary parenchymal disease in this case.

■ Essential Facts

- ASD is the most common congenital cardiac defect in adults.
- Spontaneous closure can occur in children.
- Ostium secundum ASD is the most common type and occurs in the center of the atrial chamber at the fossa ovalis.
- Ostium primum ASD occurs in the lower end of the septum inferior to the fossa ovalis. It commonly coexists with a cleft mitral valve.
- Sinus venosus ASD is uncommon and results from a defect of the superior inlet portion of the atrial septum. It is superior to the fossa ovalis near the entrance of the superior vena cava (SVC). Ninety percent of patients have partial anomalous pulmonary venous return of the right upper lobe to the SVC.
- After birth, the physiologic increase in left atrial pressure creates a left-to-right shunt. Volume overload, right heart failure, and pulmonary hypertension can develop.
- Transcatheter percutaneous closure with a septal occluder is the treatment of choice.

■ Other Imaging Findings

- Increased pulmonary blood flow is usually visible radiographically when the ratio of pulmonary to systemic blood flow is higher than 2.
- Echocardiography is the primary imaging modality for the diagnosis of ASD.
- Phase-contrast cine magnetic resonance imaging (MRI) allows quantification of the degree of shunting.
- A secundum ASD is necessary for survival in tricuspid atresia, total anomalous pulmonary venous return, and hypoplastic left heart syndrome.

✓ Pearls & ✗ Pitfalls

- ✓ Holt-Oram syndrome (heart-hand syndrome) is a familial form of ASD or ventricular septal defect associated with upper extremity anomalies.
- ✗ On MRI, the fossa ovalis may be thin and exhibit little signal intensity, leading to a misdiagnosis of ostium secundum ASD. In a true ASD, the edge of the adjacent septum should be thickened.
- ✗ The chest radiograph may be normal in cases with small shunts.

Case 96

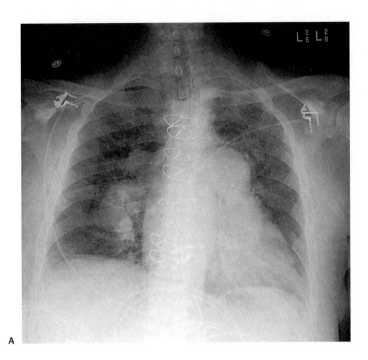

A

■ Clinical Presentation

A 45-year-old woman with dyspnea and a heart murmur.

Further Work-up

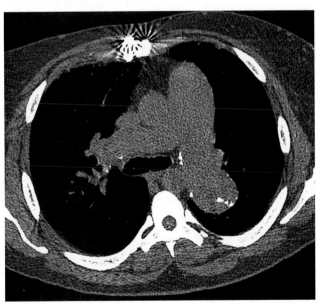

B

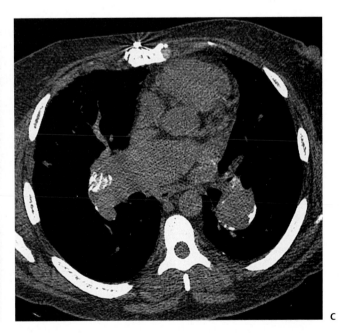

C

■ Imaging Findings

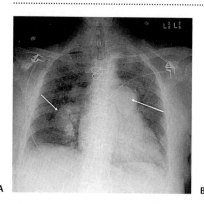
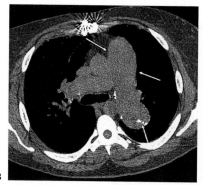
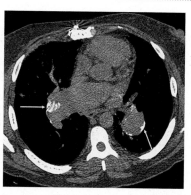

(A) Posteroanterior chest radiograph demonstrates severe enlargement of the main and central pulmonary arteries (*arrows*). **(B)** Noncontrast computed tomography (CT; lung windows) at the level of the main pulmonary artery shows significant enlargement of the pulmonary artery. Note the size discrepancy in comparison with the aorta. There is peripheral calcification involving the wall of the left pulmonary artery (*arrows*). **(C)** Noncontrast CT (lung windows) at the level of the right pulmonary artery demonstrates extensive calcification involving the walls of the pulmonary arteries bilaterally. There is a large focus of intraluminal calcification in the right main pulmonary artery (*arrows*).

■ Differential Diagnosis

- **Eisenmenger syndrome:** The findings of pulmonary artery enlargement associated with mural calcification suggest long-standing pulmonary hypertension. In this case, the patient had an atrial septal defect (not shown).
- *Pulmonary valve stenosis:* Pulmonary artery enlargement is usually isolated to the main and left pulmonary arteries.
- *Cor pulmonale:* Cor pulmonale refers to pulmonary hypertension and right ventricular dysfunction (usually hypertrophy) as the result of a respiratory disorder. There is no evidence of pulmonary parenchymal disease in this case.

■ Essential Facts

- Eisenmenger syndrome occurs in patients with large congenital intracardiac shunts. Initially, a right-to-left shunt causes increased pulmonary blood flow. With time, exposure to high pressures and flow causes morphologic changes in the vasculature, progressive elevation in the pulmonary vascular resistance, and ultimately reversal of the shunt.
- It usually develops before puberty; patients can present with reduced exercise tolerance, fatigue, dyspnea, subtle neurologic abnormalities, and/or congestive heart failure.

- It most commonly is the result of a large ventricular septal defect.
- Radiographs demonstrate dilated central pulmonary arteries and right-sided cardiac enlargement.
- There is pruning of peripheral pulmonary arteries.
- The pulmonary veins are typically not distended.
- Linear mural calcification and thrombus in the central pulmonary arteries occur with long-standing disease.
- Hypertrophic osteoarthropathy may occur.

✓ Pearls & ✗ Pitfalls

✓ The incidence of pulmonary artery thrombus formation in Eisenmenger syndrome is high.

✓ It can also occur in surgically created extracardiac left-to-right shunts.

✗ Maternal mortality rates, predominantly in the postpartum period, are high (approaching 50%) in patients with Eisenmenger syndrome, and pregnancy is contraindicated. Fetal mortality is also significantly increased.

Case 97

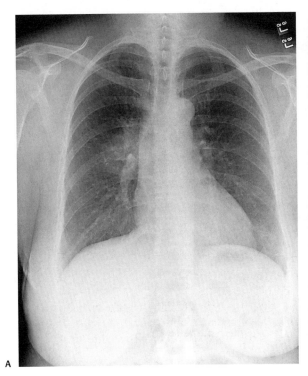

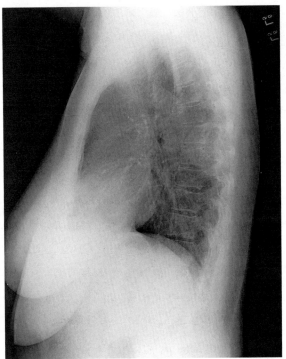

A   B

■ Clinical Presentation

A 30-year-old woman with cough.

Further Work-up

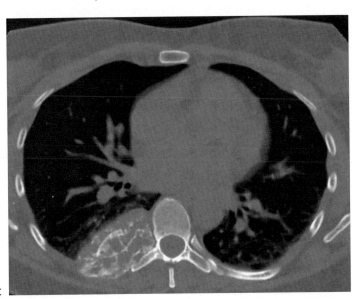

C

■ Imaging Findings

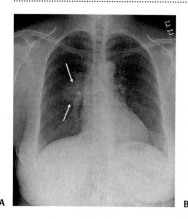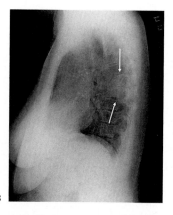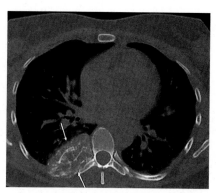

(A) Posteroanterior chest radiograph demonstrates an ill-defined opacity in the right hemithorax. The medial right 8th rib is poorly visualized (*arrows*). **(B)** Lateral chest radiograph confirms that the lesion is centered on the chest wall (*arrows*). **(C)** Noncontrast computed tomography of the chest (bone windows) shows an expansile lytic medullary lesion of the medial right 8th rib (*arrows*).

■ Differential Diagnosis

- *Fibrous dysplasia:* Although the typical "ground-glass matrix" is difficult to appreciate in this case, the findings are most consistent with fibrous dysplasia.
- *Enchondroma:* This results in focal rib expansion and may manifest typical chondroid calcification ("rings and arcs"). It rarely occurs in the ribs.
- *Ewing sarcoma:* This is typically a large mass with bone destruction seen in an adolescent.

■ Essential Facts

- Fibrous dysplasia is a developmental skeletal anomaly that usually occurs by the age of 30 years.
- Patients are usually asymptomatic.
- It is the most common benign lesion of the ribs.
- The rib cage is a common site of involvement. The craniofacial bones, femurs, and tibiae are also commonly affected.
- Fibrous dysplasia results in fusiform enlargement and deformity and loss of the normal trabecular pattern.
- The cortex is thin but preserved. Long-segment involvement is common.
- Amorphous calcification can be seen.

■ Other Imaging Findings

- Fibrous dysplasia typically shows uptake on bone scan and positron emission tomography.
- There is high or mixed signal on T2-weighted magnetic resonance imaging.

✓ Pearls & ✗ Pitfalls

- ✓ Polyostotic fibrous dysplasia has a lower prevalence. There is a homolateral distribution. When associated with mucocutaneous pigmentation and precocious puberty, it is known as McCune-Albright syndrome. When associated with fibrous and myxomatous soft-tissue tumors, it is known as Mazabraud syndrome.
- ✓ Fibrous dysplasia and osteochondroma account for most benign rib masses.
- ✗ One percent of lesions undergo malignant degeneration.

Case 98

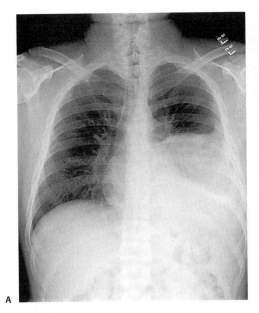

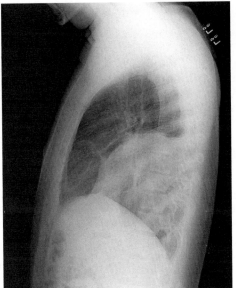

A

B

■ Clinical Presentation

An 18-year-old man with left-sided pleuritic chest pain.

Further Work-up

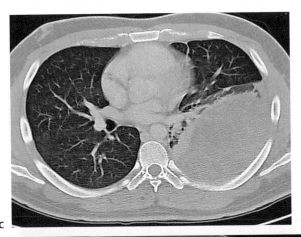

C

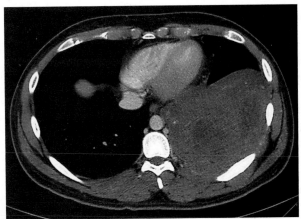

D

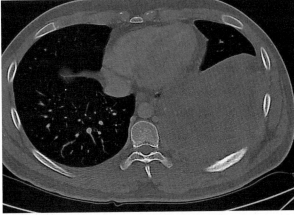

E

■ Imaging Findings

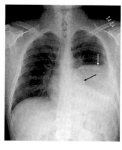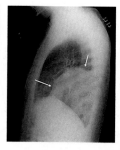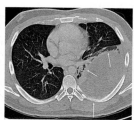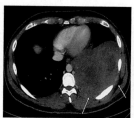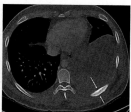

A–E

(A) Posteroanterior chest radiograph demonstrates a large mass in the left hemithorax (*white arrow*). The diaphragmatic silhouette is lost, although a portion of the left border of the heart is still seen, suggesting a posterobasal location (*black arrow*). **(B)** Lateral chest radiograph confirms the posterior location of the mass (*arrows*). There is no clear spinal or rib abnormality, although the large size of the mass makes it difficult to localize the lesion to the lung parenchyma, posterior mediastinum, or chest wall. **(C)** Contrast-enhanced computed tomography (CT) of the chest (lung windows) suggests an extrapulmonary location, given the observed mass effect (*arrows*). A left pleural effusion is present. **(D)** Contrast-enhanced CT (soft-tissue windows) demonstrates the heterogeneous density of the lesion. Note the chest wall invasion and rib sclerosis (*arrows*). **(E)** Contrast-enhanced CT (bone windows) shows the osseous involvement to advantage (*arrows*).

■ Differential Diagnosis

- *Ewing sarcoma:* A large mass of the chest wall in a patient of this age is suggestive of a sarcoma.
- *Lymphoma:* This manifests as a homogeneous pleural mass without rib destruction. There are usually other sites of disease.
- *Neuroblastoma:* This is a posterior mediastinal mass, often with calcifications. Patients are typically younger than 2 years of age.

■ Essential Facts

- The Ewing sarcoma family of tumors includes Ewing sarcoma, peripheral primitive neuroectodermal tumor, neuroepithelioma, and Askin tumor. They have a similar cellular physiology and the same reciprocal translocation of chromosomes 11 and 22.
- The tumors typically occur in children and adolescents and present with pain.
- Chest radiography demonstrates a large unilateral extrapulmonary mass.
- Rib destruction is seen in approximately two-thirds of cases.
- A pleural effusion is common.
- Lung and bone metastases can be seen in 10% of cases at presentation.
- Mass effect on the lung, or frank invasion of the pulmonary parenchyma, can occur.

■ Other Imaging Findings

- Heterogeneous signal intensity on magnetic resonance imaging is due to hemorrhage and necrosis; there is avid contrast enhancement.

✓ Pearls & ✗ Pitfalls

- ✓ Ewing sarcoma is far more common in Caucasian patients.
- ✓ It usually occurs in the ribs, scapulae, sternum, or clavicles, but extraskeletal sites of origin have been described. The neoplasm is thought to develop from embryonal neural crest cells.
- ✗ It can be difficult to determine if the mass arises from the chest wall or the pleura.

Case 99

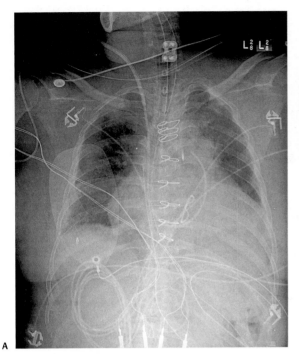

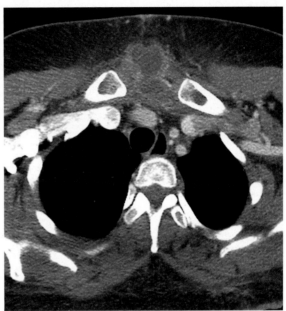

Clinical Presentation

A 52-year-old woman with fever 3 weeks after cardiac valve replacement.

Further Work-up

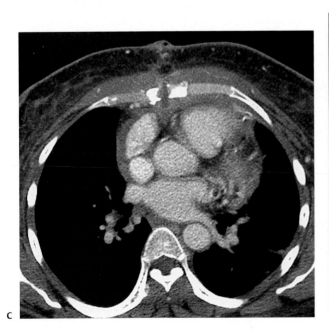

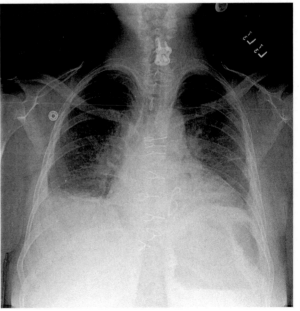

◼ Imaging Findings

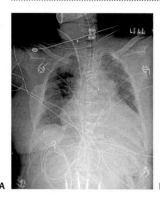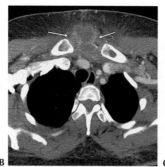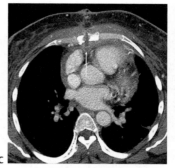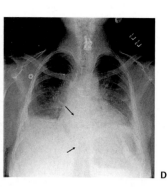

A · · · · · · · · · · · · B · · · · · · · · · · · · C · · · · · · · · · · · · D

(A) Frontal chest radiograph demonstrates displacement of multiple sternal wires. The lungs are hypoinflated, and linear atelectasis is seen at the lung bases. **(B)** Contrast-enhanced computed tomography (CT) of the chest (soft-tissue windows) through the upper sternum demonstrates a sternal abscess (*arrows*). **(C)** Contrast-enhanced CT of the chest (soft-tissue windows) through the lower sternum shows sternal nonunion with extension of the abscess into the anterior mediastinum. Note the fat stranding and pericardial effusion (*arrow*). **(D)** Frontal chest radiograph in the immediate postoperative period shows normal orientation of the sternal wires (*arrows*).

◼ Differential Diagnosis

- ***Sternal dehiscence with abscess and mediastinitis:*** Newly displaced sternal wires in association with a large fluid collection and soft-tissue stranding in the anterior mediastinum make sternal dehiscence with abscess and mediastinitis the best answer.
- *Seroma:* In the first 14 days following surgery, a fluid collection may be seen normally. The time frame and associated findings in this case make a simple fluid collection unlikely.
- *Tuberculosis (TB):* Involvement of the chest wall in TB is uncommon, although when it is present, chest wall abscess and sinus tract formation are seen in 25% of cases. These would be highly unlikely to manifest as a postoperative complication.

◼ Essential Facts

- Poststernotomy complications occur in fewer than 5% of cases.
- The mortality rate of sternal wound infection with mediastinitis is greater than 50%.
- Sternal dehiscence, mediastinitis, and osteomyelitis are the most notable poststernotomy complications.
- Complications usually manifest 1 to 2 weeks after surgery.
- Localized mediastinal fluid and pneumomediastinum are sensitive but nonspecific for mediastinitis in the first 14 days after surgery. The specificity increases significantly after 14 days.

- Sternal dehiscence is defined as complete separation of the sternum and is frequently associated with infection, most often with *Staphylococcus aureus*.
- In sternal dehiscence, the wires are typically displaced. Rotation and disruption of the wires can also occur.
- Debridement and flap closure are usually necessary.
- Following chest tube removal, there may be spontaneous evacuation of sterile fluid from the surgical site.

✓ Pearls & ✗ Pitfalls

- ✓ The term *wandering wires* has been used to describe the characteristic radiographic appearance of sternal wires in dehiscence.
- ✗ Sternal wire fracture by itself is usually not clinically significant.

Case 100

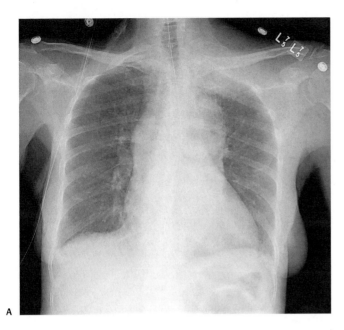

A

Clinical Presentation

A 72-year-old woman who is a smoker with shoulder pain.

Further Work-up

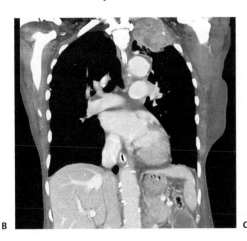

B

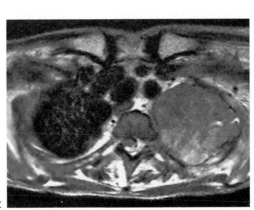

C

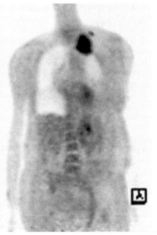

D

■ Imaging Findings

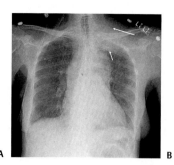 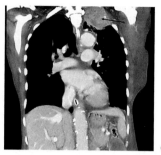 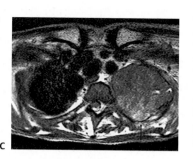 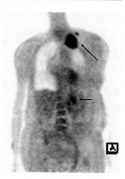

A   B   C   D

(A) Chest radiograph demonstrates a left apical mass with destruction of the first rib (*arrows*). **(B)** Coronal computed tomography (CT) reconstruction (soft-tissue windows) shows the mass to advantage (*arrow*). **(C)** Axial T2-weighted magnetic resonance imaging (MRI) shows a large left apical mass of heterogeneous signal intensity. There is chest wall invasion (*arrow*), but no encroachment on the spinal cord. **(D)** Coronal positron emission tomography (PET) scan documents the highly fluorodeoxyglucose-avid mass in the left apex (*upper arrow*). Note the adjacent hypermetabolic lymph node and left adrenal gland metastasis (*lower arrow*).

■ Differential Diagnosis

- **Superior sulcus tumor:** An apical mass with rib destruction in a patient of this age makes superior sulcus tumor the best choice. The PET scan findings demonstrate metastatic disease.
- *Tuberculosis (TB):* Reactivation TB can present as an apical lung mass, although typically other findings, such as bronchiectasis, cavitation, and scarring, are also present. Calcification may be present. Rib destruction can be associated with TB, although not as commonly as with malignancy. TB can be hypermetabolic on PET.
- *Nerve sheath tumor:* This is the most common cause of a posterior mediastinal mass. It can extend over the lung apex. Widening of the neural foramen would be expected. Frank rib destruction would not be expected.

■ Essential Facts

- Superior sulcus tumor is non–small-cell lung carcinoma arising from the lung apex and invading the chest wall or soft tissues of the thoracic inlet.
- It can be associated with Pancoast syndrome, which was originally described as shoulder and arm pain, atrophy of the hand muscles, and Horner syndrome (ptosis, miosis, anhidrosis) in association with an apical lung mass. Because not all cases of apical lung tumor result in Pancoast syndrome, the term *superior sulcus tumor* is preferred.
- Superior sulcus tumors account for 3% of primary lung cancers, with adenocarcinomas and squamous cell carcinomas accounting for most cases.

- Because the tumors are peripheral, the usual symptoms of lung cancer may be absent. Patients may present with shoulder pain or other musculoskeletal or neurologic complaints.
- An asymmetric apical cap with a convex margin of more than 5 mm, especially if it has increased in comparison with previous radiographs, is suggestive of a superior sulcus tumor.
- Osseous destruction is seen in one-third of cases.
- A lordotic radiograph may better depict the lung apex.
- On CT, rib destruction and the encasement of nerves or blood vessels are signs of chest wall invasion.
- MRI is more accurate for evaluating brachial plexus and subclavian artery involvement. Spinal extension is also usually better depicted. Cardiac and respiratory gating can be used to minimize motion and pulsation artifacts.
- Superior sulcus tumors are at least stage IIB because of extrathoracic soft-tissue invasion.

✓ Pearls & ✗ Pitfalls

- ✓ Brachial plexus invasion above T1, vertebral body invasion of more than 50%, invasion of the esophagus or trachea, distant metastases, and N2/N3 nodal metastases are considered absolute contraindications to surgical resection.
- ✓ Because T1 sagittal sequences often provide the most information, these should be performed first in case the study cannot be completed.
- ✗ In patients who have undergone resection, a cerebrospinal fluid leak due to a subarachnoid-pleural fistula may develop.
- ✗ Superior sulcus tumor is often missed on initial chest radiographs.

Further Readings

Case 1

Berrocal T, Madrid C, Novo S, Gutiérrez J, Arjonilla A, Gómez-León N. Congenital anomalies of the tracheobronchial tree, lung, and mediastinum: embryology, radiology, and pathology. Radiographics 2004;24(1):e17

Bolca N, Topal U, Bayram S. Bronchopulmonary sequestration: radiologic findings. Eur J Radiol 2004;52(2):185–191

Evrard V, Ceulemans J, Coosemans W, et al. Congenital parenchymatous malformations of the lung. World J Surg 1999;23(11):1123–1132

Zylak CJ, Eyler WR, Spizarny DL, Stone CH. Developmental lung anomalies in the adult: radiologic-pathologic correlation. Radiographics 2002;22(Spec No):S25–S43

Case 2

Berrocal T, Madrid C, Novo S, Gutiérrez J, Arjonilla A, Gómez-León N. Congenital anomalies of the tracheobronchial tree, lung, and mediastinum: embryology, radiology, and pathology. Radiographics 2004;24(1):e17

Jeung M-Y, Gasser B, Gangi A, et al. Imaging of cystic masses of the mediastinum. Radiographics 2002;22(Spec No):S79–S93

Zylak CJ, Eyler WR, Spizarny DL, Stone CH. Developmental lung anomalies in the adult: radiologic-pathologic correlation. Radiographics 2002;22(Spec No):S25–S43

Case 3

Buscarini E, Buscarini L, Civardi G, Arruzzoli S, Bossalini G, Piantanida M. Hepatic vascular malformations in hereditary hemorrhagic telangiectasia: imaging findings. AJR Am J Roentgenol 1994;163(5):1105–1110

Cottin V, Plauchu H, Bayle JY, Barthelet M, Revel D, Cordier JF. Pulmonary arteriovenous malformations in patients with hereditary hemorrhagic telangiectasia. Am J Respir Crit Care Med 2004;169(9):994–1000

Maillard J-O, Cottin V, Etienne-Mastroïanni B, Frolet JM, Revel D, Cordier JF. Pulmonary varix mimicking pulmonary arteriovenous malformation in a patient with Turner syndrome. Respiration 2007;74(1):110–113

Matsuo M, Kanematsu M, Kato H, Kondo H, Sugisaki K, Hoshi H. Osler-Weber-Rendu disease: visualizing portovenous shunting with three-dimensional sonography. AJR Am J Roentgenol 2001;176(4):919–920

Case 4

Marshall KW, Blane CE, Teitelbaum DH, van Leeuwen K. Congenital cystic adenomatoid malformation: impact of prenatal diagnosis and changing strategies in the treatment of the asymptomatic patient. AJR Am J Roentgenol 2000;175(6):1551–1554

Paterson A. Imaging evaluation of congenital lung abnormalities in infants and children. Radiol Clin North Am 2005;43(2):303–323

Restrepo S, Villamil MA, Rojas IC, et al. Association of two respiratory congenital anomalies: tracheal diverticulum and cystic adenomatoid malformation of the lung. Pediatr Radiol 2004;34(3):263–266

Stocker JT, Madewell JE, Drake RM. Congenital cystic adenomatoid malformation of the lung. Classification and morphologic spectrum. Hum Pathol 1977;8(2):155–171

Williams HJ, Johnson KJ. Imaging of congenital cystic lung lesions. Paediatr Respir Rev 2002;3(2):120–127

Case 5

Apostolopoulou SC, Kelekis NL, Brountzos EN, Rammos S, Kelekis DA. "Absent" pulmonary artery in one adult and five pediatric patients: imaging, embryology, and therapeutic implications. AJR Am J Roentgenol 2002;179(5):1253–1260

Davis SD. Case 28: Proximal interruption of the right pulmonary artery. Radiology 2000;217(2):437–440

Ryu DS, Spirn PW, Trotman-Dickenson B, et al. HRCT findings of proximal interruption of the right pulmonary artery. J Thorac Imaging 2004;19(3):171–175

Ten Harkel AD, Blom NA, Ottenkamp J. Isolated unilateral absence of a pulmonary artery: a case report and review of the literature. Chest 2002;122(4):1471–1477

Case 6

Erasmus JJ, Connolly JE, McAdams HP, Roggli VL. Solitary pulmonary nodules: Part I. Morphologic evaluation for differentiation of benign and malignant lesions. Radiographics 2000;20(1):43–58

Gould MK, Fletcher J, Iannettoni MD, et al; American College of Chest Physicians. Evaluation of patients with pulmonary nodules: when is it lung cancer?: ACCP evidence-based clinical practice guidelines (2nd edition). Chest 2007; 132(3, Suppl):108S–130S

Jeong YJ, Yi CA, Lee KS. Solitary pulmonary nodules: detection, characterization, and guidance for further diagnostic workup and treatment. AJR Am J Roentgenol 2007;188(1):57–68

MacMahon H, Austin JH, Gamsu G, et al; Fleischner Society. Guidelines for management of small pulmonary nodules detected on CT scans: a statement from the Fleischner Society. Radiology 2005;237(2):395–400

Case 7

American Thoracic Society; European Respiratory Society. American Thoracic Society/European Respiratory Society statement: standards for the diagnosis and management of individuals with alpha-1 antitrypsin deficiency. Am J Respir Crit Care Med 2003;168(7):818–900

King MA, Stone JA, Diaz PT, Mueller CF, Becker WJ, Gadek JE. Alpha1-antitrypsin deficiency: evaluation of bronchiectasis with CT. Radiology 1996;199(1):137–141

Needham M, Stockley RA. Alpha1-antitrypsin deficiency. 3: Clinical manifestations and natural history. Thorax 2004;59(5):441–445

Shaker SB, Stavngaard T, Stolk J, Stoel B, Dirksen A. Alpha1-antitrypsin deficiency. 7: Computed tomographic imaging in alpha1-antitrypsin deficiency. Thorax 2004;59(11):986–991

Case 8

Arcasoy SM, Jett JR. Superior pulmonary sulcus tumors and Pancoast's syndrome. N Engl J Med 1997;337(19):1370–1376

Attar S, Krasna MJ, Sonett JR, et al. Superior sulcus (Pancoast) tumor: experience with 105 patients. Ann Thorac Surg 1998;66(1):193–198

Bruzzi JF, Komaki R, Walsh GL, et al. Imaging of non-small cell lung cancer of the superior sulcus: part 1: anatomy, clinical manifestations, and management. Radiographics 2008;28(2):551–560, quiz 620

Bruzzi JF, Komaki R, Walsh GL, et al. Imaging of non-small cell lung cancer of the superior sulcus: part 2: initial staging and assessment of resectability and therapeutic response. Radiographics 2008;28(2):561–572

Case 9

Irshad A, Ravenel JG. Imaging of small-cell lung cancer. Curr Probl Diagn Radiol 2004;33(5):200–211

Kamel EM, Zwahlen D, Wyss MT, Stumpe KD, von Schulthess GK, Steinert HC. Whole-body (18)F-FDG PET improves the management of patients with small cell lung cancer. J Nucl Med 2003;44(12):1911–1917

Stupp R, Monnerat C, Turrisi AT III, Perry MC, Leyvraz S. Small cell lung cancer: state of the art and future perspectives. Lung Cancer 2004;45(1):105–117

Case 10

Heyneman LE, Patz EF. PET imaging in patients with bronchioloalveolar cell carcinoma. Lung Cancer 2002;38(3):261–266

Jung JI, Kim H, Park SH, et al. CT differentiation of pneumonic-type bronchioloalveolar cell carcinoma and infectious pneumonia. Br J Radiol 2001;74(882):490–494

Kim TH, Kim SJ, Ryu YH, et al. Differential CT features of infectious pneumonia versus bronchioloalveolar carcinoma (BAC) mimicking pneumonia. Eur Radiol 2006;16(8):1763–1768

Read WL, Page NC, Tierney RM, Piccirillo JF, Govindan R. The epidemiology of bronchioloalveolar carcinoma over the past two decades: analysis of the SEER database. Lung Cancer 2004;45(2):137–142

Shah RM, Miller W Jr. Widespread ground-glass opacity of the lung in consecutive patients undergoing CT: Does lobular distribution assist diagnosis? AJR Am J Roentgenol 2003;180(4):965–968

Case 11

Castañer E, Gallardo X, Rimola J, et al. Congenital and acquired pulmonary artery anomalies in the adult: radiologic overview. Radiographics 2006;26(2):349–371

Keeling AN, Costello R, Lee MJ. Rasmussen's aneurysm: a forgotten entity? Cardiovasc Intervent Radiol 2008;31(1):196–200

Nguyen ET, Silva CIS, Seely JM, Chong S, Lee KS, Müller NL. Pulmonary artery aneurysms and pseudoaneurysms in adults: findings at CT and radiography. AJR Am J Roentgenol 2007;188(2):W126–W134

Picard C, Parrot A, Boussaud V, et al. Massive hemoptysis due to Rasmussen aneurysm: detection with helicoidal CT angiography and successful steel coil embolization. Intensive Care Med 2003;29(10):1837–1839

Case 12

Aquino SL, Gamsu G, Webb WR, Kee ST. Tree-in-bud pattern: frequency and significance on thin section CT. J Comput Assist Tomogr 1996;20(4):594–599

Eisenhuber E. The tree-in-bud sign. Radiology 2002;222(3):771–772

Rossi SE, Franquet T, Volpacchio M, Giménez A, Aguilar G. Tree-in-bud pattern at thin-section CT of the lungs: radiologic-pathologic overview. Radiographics 2005;25(3):789–801

Case 13

Franquet T, Müller NL, Giménez A, Guembe P, de La Torre J, Bagué S. Spectrum of pulmonary aspergillosis: histologic, clinical, and radiologic findings. Radiographics 2001;21(4):825–837

Lynch DA. Imaging of asthma and allergic bronchopulmonary mycosis. Radiol Clin North Am 1998;36(1):129–142

Martinez S, Heyneman LE, McAdams HP, Rossi SE, Restrepo CS, Eraso A. Mucoid impactions: finger-in-glove sign and other CT and radiographic features. Radiographics 2008;28(5):1369–1382

Moss RB. Pathophysiology and immunology of allergic bronchopulmonary aspergillosis. Med Mycol 2005;43(Suppl 1):S203–S206

Case 14

Lipchik RJ, Kuzo RS. Nosocomial pneumonia. Radiol Clin North Am 1996;34(1):47–58

Moon WK, Im JG, Yeon KM, Han MC. Complications of Klebsiella pneumonia: CT evaluation. J Comput Assist Tomogr 1995;19(2):176–181

Schmidt AJ, Stark P. Radiographic findings in Klebsiella (Friedlander's) pneumonia: the bulging fissure sign. Semin Respir Infect 1998;13(1):80–82

Case 15

Alanezi M. Varicella pneumonia in adults: 13 years' experience with review of literature. Ann Thorac Med 2007;2(4):163–165

Chong S, Lee KS, Kim TS, Chung MJ, Chung MP, Han J. Adenovirus pneumonia in adults: radiographic and high-resolution CT findings in five patients. AJR Am J Roentgenol 2006;186(5):1288–1293

Kim EA, Lee KS, Primack SL, et al. Viral pneumonias in adults: radiologic and pathologic findings. Radiographics 2002;22(Spec No):S137–S149

Moon JH, Kim EA, Lee KS, Kim TS, Jung KJ, Song JH. Cytomegalovirus pneumonia: high-resolution CT findings in ten non-AIDS immunocompromised patients. Korean J Radiol 2000;1(2):73–78

Virkki R, Juven T, Rikalainen H, Svedström E, Mertsola J, Ruuskanen O. Differentiation of bacterial and viral pneumonia in children. Thorax 2002;57(5):438–441

Case 16

Boiselle PM, Crans CA Jr, Kaplan MA. The changing face of Pneumocystis carinii pneumonia in AIDS patients. AJR Am J Roentgenol 1999;172(5):1301–1309

Datta D, Ali SA, Henken EM, Kellet H, Brown S, Metersky ML. Pneumocystis carinii pneumonia: the time course of clinical and radiographic improvement. Chest 2003;124(5):1820–1823

Franquet T, Giménez A, Hidalgo A. Imaging of opportunistic fungal infections in immunocompromised patient. Eur J Radiol 2004;51(2):130–138

Saxena AK, Agarwal R. It is time to move: Pneumocystis jirovecii, not Pneumocystis carinii. Radiology 2008;246(3):985, author reply 985

Vogel MN, Brodoefel H, Hierl T, et al. Differences and similarities of cytomegalovirus and pneumocystis pneumonia in HIV-negative immunocompromised patients thin section CT morphology in the early phase of the disease. Br J Radiol 2007;80(955):516–523

Case 17

Godwin JD, Webb WR, Savoca CJ, Gamsu G, Goodman PC. Multiple, thin-walled cystic lesions of the lung. AJR Am J Roentgenol 1980;135(3):593–604

Kramer SS, Wehunt WD, Stocker JT, Kashima H. Pulmonary manifestations of juvenile laryngotracheal papillomatosis. AJR Am J Roentgenol 1985;144(4):687–694

Lui D, Kumar A, Aggarwal S, Soto J. CT findings of malignant change in recurrent respiratory papillomatosis. J Comput Assist Tomogr 1995;19(5):804–807

Restrepo S, Palacios E, Mastrogiovanni L, Kaplan J, Gordillo H. Recurrent respiratory papillomatosis. Ear Nose Throat J 2003;82(8):555–556

Soldatski IL, Onufrieva EK, Steklov AM, Schepin NV. Tracheal, bronchial, and pulmonary papillomatosis in children. Laryngoscope 2005;115(10):1848–1854

Case 18

Aquino SL, Kee ST, Warnock ML, Gamsu G. Pulmonary aspergillosis: imaging findings with pathologic correlation. AJR Am J Roentgenol 1994;163(4):811–815

Franquet T, Müller NL, Giménez A, Guembe P, de La Torre J, Bagué S. Spectrum of pulmonary aspergillosis: histologic, clinical, and radiologic findings. Radiographics 2001;21(4):825–837

Pinto PS. The CT halo sign. Radiology 2004;230(1):109–110

Sonnet S, Buitrago-Téllez CH, Tamm M, Christen S, Steinbrich W. Direct detection of angioinvasive pulmonary aspergillosis in immunosuppressed patients: preliminary results with high-resolution 16-MDCT angiography. AJR Am J Roentgenol 2005;184(3):746–751

Case 19

Gillams AR, Chaddha B, Carter AP. MR appearances of the temporal evolution and resolution of infectious spondylitis. AJR Am J Roentgenol 1996;166(4):903–907

Kapeller P, Fazekas F, Krametter D, et al. Pyogenic infectious spondylitis: clinical, laboratory and MRI features. Eur Neurol 1997;38(2):94–98

Karadimas EJ, Bunger C, Lindblad BE, et al. Spondylodiscitis. A retrospective study of 163 patients. Acta Orthop 2008;79(5):650–659

Moorthy S, Prabhu NK. Spectrum of MR imaging findings in spinal tuberculosis. AJR Am J Roentgenol 2002;179(4):979–983

Smith AS, Weinstein MA, Mizushima A, et al. MR imaging characteristics of tuberculous spondylitis vs vertebral osteomyelitis. AJR Am J Roentgenol 1989;153(2):399–405

Case 20

Boiselle PM, Mansilla AV, White CS, Fisher MS. Sternal dehiscence in patients with and without mediastinitis. J Thorac Imaging 2001;16(2):106–110

Doyle AJ, Large SR, Murphy F. Sternal wound dehiscence after internal mammary artery harvesting. Logical management. Part 2. Interact Cardiovasc Thorac Surg 2005;4(6):511–513

Li AE, Fishman EK. Evaluation of complications after sternotomy using single- and multidetector CT with three-dimensional volume rendering. AJR Am J Roentgenol 2003;181(4):1065–1070

Losanoff JE, Richman BW, Jones JW. Disruption and infection of median sternotomy: a comprehensive review. Eur J Cardiothorac Surg 2002;21(5):831–839

Case 21

Bae YA, Lee KS. Cross-sectional evaluation of thoracic lymphoma. Radiol Clin North Am 2008;46(2):253–264, viii

Duwe BV, Sterman DH, Musani AI. Tumors of the mediastinum. Chest 2005;128(4):2893–2909

Rademaker J. Hodgkin's and non-Hodgkin's lymphomas. Radiol Clin North Am 2007;45(1):69–83

Case 22

Chughtai A, Cronin P, Kelly AM, Kazerooni EA. Lung transplantation imaging in the adult. Semin Roentgenol 2006;41(1):26–35

Gotway MB, Dawn SK, Sellami D, et al. Acute rejection following lung transplantation: limitations in accuracy of thin-section CT for diagnosis. Radiology 2001;221(1):207–212

Krishnam MS, Suh RD, Tomasian A, et al. Postoperative complications of lung transplantation: radiologic findings along a time continuum. Radiographics 2007;27(4):957–974

Ng YL, Paul N, Patsios D, et al. Imaging of lung transplantation: review. AJR Am J Roentgenol 2009;192(3, Suppl):S1–S13, quiz S14–S19

Ravenel J, McAdams P. Imaging of lung transplantation. Appl Radiol 2006;35:8–20

Case 23

Buckley J, Shaw PJ, Cartledge JD, Miller RF. Multicentric plasma cell variant Castleman's disease mimicking intrapulmonary malignancy. Sex Transm Infect 2002;78(4):304–305

Guihot A, Couderc LJ, Agbalika F, et al. Pulmonary manifestations of multicentric Castleman's disease in HIV infection: a clinical, biological and radiological study. Eur Respir J 2005;26(1):118–125

Hillier JC, Shaw P, Miller RF, et al. Imaging features of multicentric Castleman's disease in HIV infection. Clin Radiol 2004;59(7):596–601

Johkoh T, Müller NL, Ichikado K, et al. Intrathoracic multicentric Castleman disease: CT findings in 12 patients. Radiology 1998;209(2):477–481

McAdams HP, Rosado-de-Christenson M, Fishback NF, Templeton PA. Castleman disease of the thorax: radiologic features with clinical and histopathologic correlation. Radiology 1998;209(1):221–228

Caser 24

Buckley J, Shaw PJ, Cartledge JD, Miller RF. Multicentric plasma cell variant Castleman's disease mimicking intrapulmonary malignancy. Sex Transm Infect 2002;78(4):304–305

Guihot A, Couderc LJ, Agbalika F, et al. Pulmonary manifestations of multicentric Castleman's disease in HIV infection: a clinical, biological and radiological study. Eur Respir J 2005;26(1):118–125

Hillier JC, Shaw P, Miller RF, et al. Imaging features of multicentric Castleman's disease in HIV infection. Clin Radiol 2004;59(7):596–601

Johkoh T, Müller NL, Ichikado K, et al. Intrathoracic multicentric Castleman disease: CT findings in 12 patients. Radiology 1998;209(2):477–481

McAdams HP, Rosado-de-Christenson M, Fishback NF, Templeton PA. Castleman disease of the thorax: radiologic features with clinical and histopathologic correlation. Radiology 1998;209(1):221–228

Case 25

Das S, Miller RF. Lymphocytic interstitial pneumonitis in HIV infected adults. Sex Transm Infect 2003;79(2):88–93

Honda O, Johkoh T, Ichikado K, et al. Differential diagnosis of lymphocytic interstitial pneumonia and malignant lymphoma on high-resolution CT. AJR Am J Roentgenol 1999;173(1):71–74

Johkoh T, Müller NL, Pickford HA, et al. Lymphocytic interstitial pneumonia: thin-section CT findings in 22 patients. Radiology 1999;212(2):567–572

Swigris JJ, Berry GJ, Raffin TA, Kuschner WG. Lymphoid interstitial pneumonia: a narrative review. Chest 2002;122(6):2150–2164

Case 26

Genofre EH, Vargas FS, Teixeira LR, et al. Reexpansion pulmonary edema. J Pneumol 2003;29(2):101–106

Hassan W, ElShaer F, Fawzy ME, Al Helaly S, Hegazy H, Akhras N. Cardiac unilateral pulmonary edema: is it really a rare presentation? Congest Heart Fail 2005;11(4):220–223

Sohara Y. Reexpansion pulmonary edema. Ann Thorac Cardiovasc Surg 2008;14(4):205–209

Young AL, Langston CS, Schiffman RL, Shortsleeve MJ. Mitral valve regurgitation causing right upper lobe pulmonary edema. Tex Heart Inst J 2001;28(1):53–56

Zegdi R, Dürrleman N, Achouh P, et al. Unilateral pulmonary edema after pulmonary embolism in a bilateral lung transplant patient. Ann Thorac Surg 2007;84(6):2086–2088

Case 27

Hagan IG, Burney K. Radiology of recreational drug abuse. Radiographics 2007;27(4):919–940

Restrepo CS, Carrillo JA, Martínez S, Ojeda P, Rivera AL, Hatta A. Pulmonary complications from cocaine and cocaine-based substances: imaging manifestations. Radiographics 2007;27(4):941–956

Restrepo CS, Rojas CA, Martínez S, et al. Cardiovascular complications of cocaine: imaging findings. Emerg Radiol 2009;16(1):11–19

Sporer KA, Dorn E. Heroin-related noncardiogenic pulmonary edema: a case series. Chest 2001;120(5):1628–1632

Sterrett C, Brownfield J, Korn CS, Hollinger M, Henderson SO. Patterns of presentation in heroin overdose resulting in pulmonary edema. Am J Emerg Med 2003;21(1):32–34

Case 28

Kim K-I, Kim CW, Lee MK, et al. Imaging of occupational lung disease. Radiographics 2001;21(6):1371–1391

OikonomouA, MullerN. Imaging of pneumoconiosis. Imaging 2003;1:11–22

Roach HD, Davies GJ, Attanoos R, Crane M, Adams H, Phillips S. Asbestos: when the dust settles an imaging review of asbestos-related disease. Radiographics 2002;22(Spec No):S167–S184

Case 29

Kim K-I, Kim CW, Lee MK, et al. Imaging of occupational lung disease. Radiographics 2001;21(6):1371–1391

Oikonomou A, Muller N. Imaging of pneumoconiosis. Imaging 2003;1:11–22

Roach HD, Davies GJ, Attanoos R, Crane M, Adams H, Phillips S. Asbestos: when the dust settles an imaging review of asbestos-related disease. Radiographics 2002;22(Spec No):S167–S184

Case 30

Bergin CJ, Müller NL, Vedal S, Chan-Yeung M. CT in silicosis: correlation with plain films and pulmonary function tests. AJR Am J Roentgenol 1986;146(3):477–483

Chong S, Lee KS, Chung MJ, Han J, Kwon OJ, Kim TS. Pneumoconiosis: comparison of imaging and pathologic findings. Radiographics 2006;26(1):59–77

Kim K-I, Kim CW, Lee MK, et al. Imaging of occupational lung disease. Radiographics 2001;21(6):1371–1391

Oikonomou A, Muller N. Imaging of pneumoconiosis. Imaging 2003;1:11–22

Ooi GC, Tsang KW, Cheung TF, et al. Silicosis in 76 men: qualitative and quantitative CT evaluation—clinical-radiologic correlation study. Radiology 2003;228(3):816–825

Case 31

Hanak V, Golbin JM, Hartman TE, Ryu JH. High-resolution CT findings of parenchymal fibrosis correlate with prognosis in hypersensitivity pneumonitis. Chest 2008;134(1):133–138

Matar LD, McAdams HP, Sporn TA. Hypersensitivity pneumonitis. AJR Am J Roentgenol 2000;174(4):1061–1066

Selman M. Hypersensitivity pneumonitis: a multifaceted deceiving disorder. Clin Chest Med 2004;25(3):531–547, vi

Silva CIS, Churg A, Müller NL. Hypersensitivity pneumonitis: spectrum of high-resolution CT and pathologic findings. AJR Am J Roentgenol 2007;188(2):334–344

Case 32

Frazier AA, Franks TJ, Cooke EO, Mohammed TL, Pugatch RD, Galvin JR. From the archives of the AFIP: pulmonary alveolar proteinosis. Radiographics 2008;28(3):883–899, quiz 915

Seymour JF, Presneill JJ. Pulmonary alveolar proteinosis: progress in the first 44 years. Am J Respir Crit Care Med 2002;166(2):215–23512119235

Trapnell BC, Whitsett JA, Nakata K. Pulmonary alveolar proteinosis. N Engl J Med 2003;349(26):2527–2539

Case 33

Baron SE, Haramati LB, Rivera VT. Radiological and clinical findings in acute and chronic exogenous lipoid pneumonia. J Thorac Imaging 2003;18(4):217–224

Franquet T, Giménez A, Bordes R, Rodríguez-Arias JM, Castella J. The crazy-paving pattern in exogenous lipoid pneumonia: CT-pathologic correlation. AJR Am J Roentgenol 1998;170(2):315–317

Gondouin A, Manzoni P, Ranfaing E, et al. Exogenous lipid pneumonia: a retrospective multicentre study of 44 cases in France. Eur Respir J 1996;9(7):1463–1469

Laurent F, Philippe JC, Vergier B, et al. Exogenous lipoid pneumonia: HRCT, MR, and pathologic findings. Eur Radiol 1999;9(6):1190–1196

Zanetti G, Marchiori E, Gasparetto TD, Escuissato DL, Soares Souza A Jr. Lipoid pneumonia in children following aspiration of mineral oil used in the treatment of constipation: high-resolution CT findings in 17 patients. Pediatr Radiol 2007;37(11):1135–1139

Case 34

Behar JV, Choi Y-W, Hartman TA, Allen NB, McAdams HP. Relapsing polychondritis affecting the lower respiratory tract. AJR Am J Roentgenol 2002;178(1):173–177

Faix LE, Branstetter BF IV. Uncommon CT findings in relapsing polychondritis. AJNR Am J Neuroradiol 2005;26(8):2134–2136

Lee KS, Ernst A, Trentham DE, Lunn W, Feller-Kopman DJ, Boiselle PM. Relapsing polychondritis: prevalence of expiratory CT airway abnormalities. Radiology 2006;240(2):565–573

Trentham DE, Le CH. Relapsing polychondritis. Ann Intern Med 1998;129(2):114–122

Case 35

Boiselle PM, Feller-Kopman D, Ashiku S, Weeks D, Ernst A. Tracheobronchomalacia: evolving role of dynamic multislice helical CT. Radiol Clin North Am 2003;41(3):627–636

Boiselle PM, Lee KS, Lin S, Raptopoulos V. Cine CT during coughing for assessment of tracheomalacia: preliminary experience with 64-MDCT. AJR Am J Roentgenol 2006;187(2):W175–W177

Carden KA, Boiselle PM, Waltz DA, Ernst A. Tracheomalacia and tracheobronchomalacia in children and adults: an in-depth review. Chest 2005;127(3):984–1005

Case 36

Cassada DC, Munyikwa MP, Moniz MP, Dieter RA Jr, Schuchmann GF, Enderson BL. Acute injuries of the trachea and major bronchi: importance of early diagnosis. Ann Thorac Surg 2000;69(5):1563–1567

Chen J-D, Shanmuganathan K, Mirvis SE, Killeen KL, Dutton RP. Using CT to diagnose tracheal rupture. AJR Am J Roentgenol 2001;176(5):1273–1280

Rollins RJ, Tocino I. Early radiographic signs of tracheal rupture. AJR Am J Roentgenol 1987;148(4):695–698

Rossbach MM, Johnson SB, Gomez MA, Sako EY, Miller OL, Calhoon JH. Management of major tracheobronchial injuries: a 28-year experience. Ann Thorac Surg 1998;65(1):182–186

Wintermark M, Schnyder P. The Macklin effect: a frequent etiology for pneumomediastinum in severe blunt chest trauma. Chest 2001;120(2):543–547

Case 37

Berdon WE. Rings, slings, and other things: vascular compression of the infant trachea updated from the midcentury to the millennium—the legacy of Robert E. Gross, MD, and Edward B. D. Neuhauser, MD. Radiology 2000;216(3):624–632

Berdon WE, Baker DH, Wung JT, et al. Complete cartilage-ring tracheal stenosis associated with anomalous left pulmonary artery: the ring-sling complex. Radiology 1984;152(1):57–64

Lee K-H, Yoon C-S, Choe KO, et al. Use of imaging for assessing anatomical relationships of tracheobronchial anomalies associated with left pulmonary artery sling. Pediatr Radiol 2001;31(4):269–278

Newman B, Meza MP, Towbin RB, Nido PD. Left pulmonary artery sling: diagnosis and delineation of associated tracheobronchial anomalies with MR. Pediatr Radiol 1996;26(9):661–668

Case 38

Balakrishnan J, Meziane MA, Siegelman SS, Fishman EK. Pulmonary infarction: CT appearance with pathologic correlation. J Comput Assist Tomogr 1989;13(6):941–945

He EE, Müller NL, Kim KI, Wiggs BR, Mayo JR. Acute pulmonary embolism: ancillary findings at spiral CT. Radiology 1998;207(3):753–758

M-P, Triki R, Chatellier G, et al. Is It possible to recognize pulmonary infarction on multisection CT images? Radiology 2007;244(3):875–882

Toshiko H, Hidekazu M, et al. CT findings of pulmonary infarction associated with lung cancer. Surgical and pathologic correlation. Lung Cancer 1998;38(7):891–896

Case 39

Cronin CG, Lohan DG, Keane M, Roche C, Murphy JM. Prevalence and significance of asymptomatic venous thromboembolic disease found on oncologic staging CT. AJR Am J Roentgenol 2007;189(1):162–170

Gladish GW, Choe DH, Marom EM, Sabloff BS, Broemeling LD, Munden RF. Incidental pulmonary emboli in oncology patients: prevalence, CT evaluation, and natural history. Radiology 2006;240(1):246–255

O'Connell CL, Boswell WD, Duddalwar V, et al. Unsuspected pulmonary emboli in cancer patients: clinical correlates and relevance. J Clin Oncol 2006;24(30):4928–4932

Sørensen HT, Mellemkjaer L, Steffensen FH, Olsen JH, Nielsen GL. The risk of a diagnosis of cancer after primary deep venous thrombosis or pulmonary embolism. N Engl J Med 1998;338(17):1169–1173

Case 40

Creasy JD, Chiles C, Routh WD, Dyer RB. Overview of traumatic injury of the thoracic aorta. Radiographics 1997;17(1):27–45

Dyer DS, Moore EE, Mestek MF, et al. Can chest CT be used to exclude aortic injury? Radiology 1999;213(1):195–202

Gavant ML, Menke PG, Fabian T, Flick PA, Graney MJ, Gold RE. Blunt traumatic aortic rupture: detection with helical CT of the chest. Radiology 1995;197(1):125–133

Mirvis SE, Shanmuganathan K, Miller BH, White CS, Turney SZ. Traumatic aortic injury: diagnosis with contrast-enhanced thoracic CT—five-year experience at a major trauma center. Radiology 1996;200(2):413–422

Case 41

Cantwell CP. The dependent viscera sign. Radiology 2006;238(2):752–753

Iochum S, Ludig T, Walter F, Sebbag H, Grosdidier G, Blum AG. Imaging of diaphragmatic injury: a diagnostic challenge? Radiographics 2002;22(Spec No):S103–S116, discussion S116–S118

Larici AR, Gotway MB, Litt HI, et al. Helical CT with sagittal and coronal reconstructions: accuracy for detection of diaphragmatic injury. AJR Am J Roentgenol 2002;179(2):451–457

Nchimi A, Szapiro D, Ghaye B, et al. Helical CT of blunt diaphragmatic rupture. AJR Am J Roentgenol 2005;184(1):24–3015615945

Worthy SA, Kang EY, Hartman TE, Kwong JS, Mayo JR, Müller NL. Diaphragmatic rupture: CT findings in 11 patients. Radiology 1995;194(3):885–888

Case 42

Cassada DC, Munyikwa MP, Moniz MP, Dieter RA Jr, Schuchmann GF, Enderson BL. Acute injuries of the trachea and major bronchi: importance of early diagnosis. Ann Thorac Surg 2000;69(5):1563–1567

Chen J-D, Shanmuganathan K, Mirvis SE, Killeen KL, Dutton RP. Using CT to diagnose tracheal rupture. AJR Am J Roentgenol 2001;176(5):1273–1280

Rollins RJ, Tocino I. Early radiographic signs of tracheal rupture. AJR Am J Roentgenol 1987;148(4):695–698

Rossbach MM, Johnson SB, Gomez MA, Sako EY, Miller OL, Calhoon JH. Management of major tracheobronchial injuries: a 28-year experience. Ann Thorac Surg 1998;65(1):182–186

Wintermark M, Schnyder P. The Macklin effect: a frequent etiology for pneumomediastinum in severe blunt chest trauma. Chest 2001;120(2):543–547

Case 43

Hiller N, Zagal I, Hadas-Halpern I. Spontaneous intramural hematoma of the esophagus. Am J Gastroenterol 1999;94(8):2282–2284

Modi P, Edwards A, Fox B, Rahamim J. Dissecting intramural haematoma of the oesophagus. Eur J Cardiothorac Surg 2005;27(1):171–173

Restrepo CS, Lemos DF, Ocazionez D, Moncada R, Gimenez CR. Intramural hematoma of the esophagus: a pictorial essay. Emerg Radiol 2008;15(1):13–22

Young CA, Menias CO, Bhalla S, Prasad SR. CT features of esophageal emergencies. Radiographics 2008;28(6):1541–1553

Case 44

Ghanem N, Altehoefer C, Springer O, et al. Radiological findings in Boerhaave's syndrome. Emerg Radiol 2003;10(1):8–13

Pate JW, Walker WA, Cole FH Jr, Owen EW, JohnsonWH. Spontaneous rupture of the esophagus: a 30-year experience. Ann Thorac Surg 1989;47(5):689–692

Younes Z, Johnson DA. The spectrum of spontaneous and iatrogenic esophageal injury: perforations, Mallory-Weiss tears, and hematomas. J Clin Gastroenterol 1999;29(4):306–317

Young CA, Menias CO, Bhalla S, Prasad SR. CT features of esophageal emergencies. Radiographics 2008;28(6):1541–1553

Case 45

Jang KM, Lee KS, Lee SJ, et al. The spectrum of benign esophageal lesions: imaging findings. Korean J Radiol 2002;3(3):199–210

Mutrie CJ, Donahue DM, Wain JC, et al. Esophageal leiomyoma: a 40-year experience. Ann Thorac Surg 2005;79(4):1122–1125

Spechler SJ, Waxman I. Esophageal leiomyomas. Curr Treat Options Gastroenterol 2000;3(1):71–76

Yang PS, Lee KS, Lee SJ, et al. Esophageal leiomyoma: radiologic findings in 12 patients. Korean J Radiol 2001;2(3):132–137

Case 46

Chauhan SS, Long JD. Managament of tracheoesophageal fistulas in adults. Curr Treat Options Gastroenterol 2004;7(1):31–40

Giménez A, Franquet T, Erasmus JJ, Martínez S, Estrada P. Thoracic complications of esophageal disorders. Radiographics 2002;22(Spec No):S247–S258

Sarper A, Oz N, Cihangir C, Demircan A, Isin E. The efficacy of self-expanding metal stents for palliation of malignant esophageal strictures and fistulas. Eur J Cardiothorac Surg 2003;23(5):794–798

Case 47

Baldt MM, Bankier AA, Germann PS, Pöschl GP, Skrbensky GT, Herold CJ. Complications after emergency tube thoracostomy: assessment with CT. Radiology 1995;195(2):539–543

Deneuville M. Morbidity of percutaneous tube thoracostomy in trauma patients. Eur J Cardiothorac Surg 2002;22(5):673–678

Swain FR, Martinez F, Gripp M, Razdan R, Gagliardi J. Traumatic complications from placement of thoracic catheters and tubes. Emerg Radiol 2005;12(1-2):11–18

Case 48

Burney K, Burchard F, Papouchado M, Wilde P. Cardiac pacing systems and implantable cardiac defibrillators (ICDs): a radiological perspective of equipment, anatomy and complications. Clin Radiol 2004;59(8):699–708

Daly BD, Cascade PN, Hummel JD, et al. Transvenous and subcutaneous implantable cardioverter defibrillators: radiographic assessment. Radiology 1994;191(1):273–278

Faris OP, Shein M. Food and Drug Administration perspective: Magnetic resonance imaging of pacemaker and implantable cardioverter-defibrillator patients. Circulation 2006;114(12):1232–1233

Harcombe AA, Newell SA, Ludman PF, et al. Late complications following permanent pacemaker implantation or elective unit replacement. Heart 1998;80(3):240–244

Kiviniemi MS, Pirnes MA, Eränen HJ, Kettunen RV, Hartikainen JE. Complications related to permanent pacemaker therapy. Pacing Clin Electrophysiol 1999;22(5):711–720

Steiner RM, Tegtmeyer CJ, Morse D, et al. The radiology of cardiac pacemakers. Radiographics 1986;6(3):373–399

Case 49

Aboulafia DM. The epidemiologic, pathologic, and clinical features of AIDS-associated pulmonary Kaposi's sarcoma. Chest 2000;117(4):1128–1145

Caponetti G, Dezube BJ, Restrepo CS, Pantanowitz L. Kaposi sarcoma of the musculoskeletal system: a review of 66 patients. Cancer 2007;109(6):1040–1052

Restrepo CS, Martínez S, Lemos JA, et al. Imaging manifestations of Kaposi sarcoma. Radiographics 2006;26(4):1169–1185

Traill ZC, Miller RF, Shaw PJ. CT appearances of intrathoracic Kaposi's sarcoma in patients with AIDS. Br J Radiol 1996;69(828):1104–1107

Wolff SD, Kuhlman JE, Fishman EK. Thoracic Kaposi sarcoma in AIDS: CT findings. J Comput Assist Tomogr 1993;17(1):60–62

Case 50

Bernard AW, Yasin Z, Venkat A. Acute chest syndrome of sickle cell disease. Hosp Physician 2007;43:15–23

Leong CS, Stark P. Thoracic manifestations of sickle cell disease. J Thorac Imaging 1998;13(2):128–134

Lonergan GJ, Cline DB, Abbondanzo SL. Sickle cell anemia. Radiographics 2001;21(4):971–994

Siddiqui AK, Ahmed S. Pulmonary manifestations of sickle cell disease. Postgrad Med J 2003;79(933):384–390

Vichinsky EP, Styles LA, Colangelo LH, Wright EC, Castro O, Nickerson B; Cooperative Study of Sickle Cell Disease. Acute chest syndrome in sickle cell disease: clinical presentation and course. Blood 1997;89(5):1787–1792

Case 51

Johkoh T, Itoh H, Müller NL, et al. Crazy-paving appearance at thin-section CT: spectrum of disease and pathologic findings. Radiology 1999;211(1):155–160

Rossi SE, Erasmus JJ, Volpacchio M, Franquet T, Castiglioni T, McAdams HP. "Crazy-paving" pattern at thin-section CT of the lungs: radiologic-pathologic overview. Radiographics 2003;23(6):1509–1519

Case 52

Ferguson EC, Krishnamurthy R, Oldham SAA. Classic imaging signs of congenital cardiovascular abnormalities. Radiographic 2007;27(5):1323–1334

Konen E, Raviv-Zilka L, Cohen RA, et al. Congenital pulmonary v bar syndrome: spectrum of helical CT findings with emphasi on computerized reformatting. Radiographics 2003;23(5):11 1184

Case 53

Lynch DA, Gamsu G, Ray CS, Aberle DR. Asbestos-related focal lung masses: manifestations on conventional and high-resolution CT scans. Radiology 1988;169(3):603–607

Partap VA. The comet tail sign. Radiology 1999;213(2):553–554

Case 54

Gupta P. The Golden S sign. Radiology 2004;233(3):790–791

Case 55

Abramson S. The air crescent sign. Radiology 2001;218(1):230–232

Franquet T, Müller NL, Giménez A, Guembe P, de La Torre J, Bagué S. Spectrum of pulmonary aspergillosis: histologic, clinical, and radiologic findings. Radiographics 2001;21(4):825–837

Pinto PS. The CT Halo Sign. Radiology 2004;230(1):109–110

Case 56

Gaerte SC, Meyer CA, Winer-Muram HT, Tarver RD, Conces DJ Jr. Fat-containing lesions of the chest. Radiographics 2002;22(Spec No):S61–S78

Jeong YJ, Yi CA, Lee KS. Solitary pulmonary nodules: detection, characterization, and guidance for further diagnostic workup and treatment. AJR Am J Roentgenol 2007;188(1):57–68

Case 57

Koyama T, Ueda H, Togashi K, Umeoka S, Kataoka M, Nagai S. Radiologic manifestations of sarcoidosis in various organs. Radiographics 2004;24(1):87–104

Miller BH, Rosado-de-Christenson ML, McAdams HP, Fishback NF. Thoracic sarcoidosis: radiologic-pathologic correlation. Radiographics 1995;15(2):421–437

Prabhakar HB, Rabinowitz CB, Gibbons FK, O'Donnell WJ, Shepard JA, Aquino SL. Imaging features of sarcoidosis on MDCT, FDG PET, and PET/CT. AJR Am J Roentgenol 2008; 190(3, Suppl):S1–S6

Traill ZC, Maskell GF, Gleeson FV, High-Resolution CT. High-resolution CT findings of pulmonary sarcoidosis. AJR Am J Roentgenol 1997;168(6):1557–1560

Case 58

Agrons GA, Rosado-de-Christenson ML, Kirejczyk WM, Conran RM, Stocker JT. Pulmonary inflammatory pseudotumor: radiologic features. Radiology 1998;206(2):511–518

Giménez A, Franquet T, Prats R, Estrada P, Villalba J, Bagué S. Unusual primary lung tumors: a radiologic-pathologic overview. Radiographics 2002;22(3):601–619

Narla LD, Newman B, Spottswood SS, Narla S, Kolli R. Inflammatory pseudotumor. Radiographics 2003;23(3):719–729

Case 59

Beama...
logic-pat...
148

Case 60

Coppage L, Shaw C, Curtis AM. Metastatic disease to the chest in patients with extrathoracic malignancy. J Thorac Imaging 1987;2(4):24–37

Seo JB, Im JG, Goo JM, Chung MJ, Kim MY. Atypical pulmonary metastases: spectrum of radiologic findings. Radiographics 2001;21(2):403–417

Case 61

Munk PL, Müller NL, Miller RR, Ostrow DN. Pulmonary lymphangitic carcinomatosis: CT and pathologic findings. Radiology 1988;166(3):705–709

Stein MG, Mayo J, Müller N, Aberle DR, Webb WR, Gamsu G. Pulmonary lymphangitic spread of carcinoma: appearance on CT scans. Radiology 1987;162(2):371–375

Webb WR. Thin-section CT of the secondary pulmonary lobule: anatomy and the image—the 2004 Fleischner lecture. Radiology 2006;239(2):322–338

Case 62

Chiles C, Woodard PK, Gutierrez FR, Link KM. Metastatic involvement of the heart and pericardium: CT and MR imaging. Radiographics 2001;21(2):439–449

Grebenc ML, Rosado de Christenson ML, Burke AP, Green CE, Galvin JR. Primary cardiac and pericardial neoplasms: radiologic-pathologic correlation. Radiographics 2000;20(4):1073–1103, quiz 1110–1111, 1112

Kim JS, Kim HH, Yoon Y. Imaging of pericardial diseases. Clin Radiol 2007;62(7):626–631

Nishino M, Hayakawa K, Minami M, Yamamoto A, Ueda H, Takasu K. Primary retroperitoneal neoplasms: CT and MR imaging findings with anatomic and pathologic diagnostic clues. Radiographics 2003;23(1):45–57

Case 63

Brown K, Mund DF, Aberle DR, Batra P, Young DA. Intrathoracic calcifications: radiographic features and differential diagnoses. Radiographics 1994;14(6):1247–1261

Seo JB, Im JG, Goo JM, Chung MJ, Kim MY. Atypical pulmonary metastases: spectrum of radiologic findings. Radiographics 2001;21(2):403–417

Case 64

Fishman EK, Kuhlman JE, Jones RJ. CT of lymphoma: spectrum of disease. Radiographics 1991;11(4):647–669

Strollo DC, Rosado de Christenson ML, Jett JR. Primary mediastinal tumors. Part 1: tumors of the anterior mediastinum. Chest 1997;112(2):511–522

Whitten CR, Khan S, Munneke GJ, Grubnic S. A diagnostic approach to mediastinal abnormalities. Radiographics 2007;27(3):657–671

Case 65

Berkmen YM, Zalta BA. Case 126: extramedullary hematopoiesis. Radiology 2007;245(3):905–908

Ejindu VC, Hine AL, Mashayekhi M, Shorvon PJ, Misra RR. Musculoskeletal manifestations of sickle cell disease. Radiographics 2007;27(4):1005–1021

Kawashima A, Fishman EK, Kuhlman JE, Nixon MS. CT of posterior mediastinal masses. Radiographics 1991;11(6):1045–1067

Pfeiffer EA, Coppage L, Conway WF. General case of the day. Extramedullary hematopoiesis (EH) in a patient with beta-thalassemia. Radiographics 1995;15(1):235–238

Whitten CR, Khan S, Munneke GJ, Grubnic S. A diagnostic approach to mediastinal abnormalities. Radiographics 2007;27(3):657–67

Case 66

Rosado-de-Christenson ML, Templeton PA, Moran CA. From the archives of the AFIP. Mediastinal germ cell tumors: radiologic and pathologic correlation. Radiographics 1992;12(5):1013–1030

Strollo DC, Rosado-de-Christenson ML. Primary mediastinal malignant germ cell neoplasms: imaging features. Chest Surg Clin N Am 2002;12(4):645–658

Whitten CR, Khan S, Munneke GJ, Grubnic S. A diagnostic approach to mediastinal abnormalities. Radiographics 2007;27(3):657–671

Case 67

Rosado-de-Christenson ML, Galobardes J, Moran CA. Thymoma: radiologic-pathologic correlation. Radiographics 1992;12(1):151–168

Whitten CR, Khan S, Munneke GJ, GrubnicS . A diagnostic approach to mediastinal abnormalities. Radiographics 2007;27(3):657–671

Case 68

Koyama T, Ueda H, Togashi K, Umeoka S, Kataoka M, Nagai S. Radiologic manifestations of sarcoidosis in various organs. Radiographics 2004;24(1):87–104

Miller BH, Rosado-de-Christenson ML, McAdams HP, Fishback NF. Thoracic sarcoidosis: radiologic-pathologic correlation. Radiographics 1995;15(2):421–437

Prabhakar HB, Rabinowitz CB, Gibbons FK, O'Donnell WJ, Shepard JA, Aquino SL. Imaging features of sarcoidosis on MDCT, FDG PET, and PET/CT. AJR Am J Roentgenol 2008; 190(3, Suppl):S1–S6

Traill ZC, Maskell GF, Gleeson FV, High-Resolution CT. High-resolution CT findings of pulmonary sarcoidosis. AJR Am J Roentgenol 1997;168(6):1557–1560

Case 69

Gallego C, Velasco M, Marcuello P, Tejedor D, De Campo L, Friera A. Congenital and acquired anomalies of the portal venous system. Radiographics 2002;22(1):141–159

Case 70

Kuhlman JE, Pozniak MA, Collins J, Knisely BL. Radiographic and CT findings of blunt chest trauma: aortic injuries and looking beyond them. Radiographics 1998;18(5):1085–1106, discussion 1107–1108, quiz 1

TocinoIM. Pneumothorax in the supine patient: radiographic anatomy. Radiographics 1985;5:557–586

Case 71

Aberle DR, Gamsu G, Lynch D. Thoracic manifestations of Wegener granulomatosis: diagnosis and course. Radiology 1990;174(3 Pt 1):703–709

Frazier AA, Rosado-de-Christenson ML, Galvin JR, Fleming MV. Pulmonary angiitis and granulomatosis: radiologic-pathologic correlation. Radiographics 1998;18(3):687–710, quiz 727

Case 72

Kim SJ, Lee KS, Ryu YH, et al. Reversed halo sign on high-resolution CT of cryptogenic organizing pneumonia: diagnostic implications. AJR Am J Roentgenol 2003;180(5):1251–1254

Lynch DA, Travis WD, Müller NL, et al. Idiopathic interstitial pneumonias: CT features. Radiology 2005;236(1):10–21

Mueller-Mang C, Grosse C, Schmid K, Stiebellehner L, Bankier AA. What every radiologist should know about idiopathic interstitial pneumonias. Radiographics 2007;27(3):595–615

Case 73

Lynch DA, Travis WD, Müller NL, et al. Idiopathic interstitial pneumonias: CT features. Radiology 2005;236(1):10–21

Mueller-Mang C, Grosse C, Schmid K, Stiebellehner L, Bankier AA. What every radiologist should know about idiopathic interstitial pneumonias. Radiographics 2007;27(3):595–615

Case 74

Lynch DA, Travis WD, Müller NL, et al. Idiopathic interstitial pneumonias: CT features. Radiology 2005;236(1):10–21

Mueller-Mang C, Grosse C, Schmid K, Stiebellehner L, Bankier AA. What every radiologist should know about idiopathic interstitial pneumonias. Radiographics 2007;27(3):595–615

Case 75

Attili AK, Kazerooni EA, Gross BH, Flaherty KR, Myers JL, Martinez FJ. Smoking-related interstitial lung disease: radiologic-clinical-pathologic correlation. Radiographics 2008;28(5):1383–1396, discussion 1396–1398

Lynch DA, Travis WD, Müller NL, et al. Idiopathic interstitial pneumonias: CT features. Radiology 2005;236(1):10–21

Mueller-Mang C, Grosse C, Schmid K, Stiebellehner L, Bankier AA. What every radiologist should know about idiopathic interstitial pneumonias. Radiographics 2007;27(3):595–615

Case 76

Kim EA, Lee KS, Johkoh T, et al. Interstitial lung diseases associated with collagen vascular diseases: radiologic and histopathologic findings. Radiographics 2002;22(Spec No):S151–S165

Mayberry JP, Primack SL, Müller NL. Thoracic manifestations of systemic autoimmune diseases: radiographic and high-resolution CT findings. Radiographics 2000;20(6):1623–1635

Case 77

Giménez A, Franquet T, Prats R, Estrada P, Villalba J, Bagué S. Unusual primary lung tumors: a radiologic-pathologic overview. Radiographics 2002;22(3):601–619

Prince JS, Duhamel DR, Levin DL, Harrell JH, Friedman PJ. Nonneoplastic lesions of the tracheobronchial wall: radiologic findings with bronchoscopic correlation. Radiographics 2002;22(Spec No):S215–S230

Case 78

Collins J, Stern EJ. Ground-glass opacity at CT: the ABCs. AJR Am J Roentgenol 1997;169(2):355–367

Lynch DA, Travis WD, Müller NL, et al. Idiopathic interstitial pneumonias: CT features. Radiology 2005;236(1):10–21

Unger JM, Peters ME, Hinke ML. Chest case of the day. AJR Am J Roentgenol 1986;146(5):1080–1086

Ware LB, Matthay MA. The acute respiratory distress syndrome. N Engl J Med 2000;342(18):1334–1349

Case 79

Koyama T, Ueda H, Togashi K, Umeoka S, Kataoka M, Nagai S. Radiologic manifestations of sarcoidosis in various organs. Radiographics 2004;24(1):87–104

Miller BH, Rosado-de-Christenson ML, McAdams HP, Fishback NF. Thoracic sarcoidosis: radiologic-pathologic correlation. Radiographics 1995;15(2):421–437

Prabhakar HB, Rabinowitz CB, Gibbons FK, O'Donnell WJ, Shepard JA, Aquino SL. Imaging features of sarcoidosis on MDCT, FDG PET, and PET/CT. AJR Am J Roentgenol 2008; 190(3, Suppl):S1–S6

Traill ZC, Maskell GF, Gleeson FV, High-Resolution CT. High-resolution CT findings of pulmonary sarcoidosis. AJR Am J Roentgenol 1997;168(6):1557–1560

Case 80

Kraus GJ. The split pleura sign. Radiology 2007;243(1):297–298

Kuhlman JE, Singha NK. Complex disease of the pleural space: radiographic and CT evaluation. Radiographics 1997;17(1):63–799

Case 81

Giménez A, Franquet T, Prats R, Estrada P, Villalba J, Bagué S. Unusual primary lung tumors: a radiologic-pathologic overview. Radiographics 2002;22(3):601–619

Prince JS, Duhamel DR, Levin DL, Harrell JH, Friedman PJ. Nonneoplastic lesions of the tracheobronchial wall: radiologic findings with bronchoscopic correlation. Radiographics 2002;22(Spec No):S215–S230

Case 82

Abbott GF, Rosado-de-Christenson ML, Franks TJ, Frazier AA, Galvin JR. From the archives of the AFIP: pulmonary Langerhans cell histiocytosis. Radiographics 2004;24(3):821–84115143231

Brauner MW, Grenier P, Tijani K, Battesti JP, Valeyre D. Pulmonary Langerhans cell histiocytosis: evolution of lesions on CT scans. Radiology 1997;204(2):497–502

Case 83

Kramer SS, Wehunt WD, Stocker JT, Kashima H. Pulmonary manifestations of juvenile laryngotracheal papillomatosis. AJR Am J Roentgenol 1985;144(4):687–694

Kuhlman JE, Reyes BL, Hruban RH, et al. Abnormal air-filled spaces in the lung. Radiographics 1993;13(1):47–75

Prince JS, Duhamel DR, Levin DL, Harrell JH, Friedman PJ. Nonneoplastic lesions of the tracheobronchial wall: radiologic findings with bronchoscopic correlation. Radiographics 2002;22(Spec No):S215–S230

Case 84

Lynch DA, Travis WD, Müller NL, et al. Idiopathic interstitial pneumonias: CT features. Radiology 2005;236(1):10–21

Mueller-Mang C, Grosse C, Schmid K, Stiebellehner L, Bankier AA. What every radiologist should know about idiopathic interstitial pneumonias. Radiographics 2007;27(3):595–615

Case 85

Erasmus JJ, McAdams HP, Farrell MA, Patz EF Jr. Pulmonary nontuberculous mycobacterial infection: radiologic manifestations. Radiographics 1999;19(6):1487–1505

Rossi SE, Franquet T, Volpacchio M, Giménez A, Aguilar G. Tree-in-bud pattern at thin-section CT of the lungs: radiologic-pathologic overview. Radiographics 2005;25(3):789–801

Wittram C, Weisbrod GL. Mycobacterium avium complex lung disease in immunocompetent patients: radiography-CT correlation. Br J Radiol 2002;75(892):340–344

Case 86

Burrill J, Williams CJ, Bain G, Conder G, Hine AL, Misra RR. Tuberculosis: a radiologic review. Radiographics 2007;27(5):1255–1273

Kato A, Kudo S, Matsumoto K, et al. Bronchial artery embolization for hemoptysis due to benign diseases: immediate and long-term results. Cardiovasc Intervent Radiol 2000;23(5):351–357

Kim HY, Song KS, Goo JM, Lee JS, Lee KS, Lim TH. Thoracic sequelae and complications of tuberculosis. Radiographics 2001;21(4):839–858, discussion 859–860

Case 87

Hartman TE, Primack SL, Lee KS, Swensen SJ, Müller NL. CT of bronchial and bronchiolar diseases. Radiographics 1994;14(5):991–1003

Nadel HR, Stringer DA, Levison H, Turner JA, Sturgess JM. The immotile cilia syndrome: radiological manifestations. Radiology 1985;154(3):651–655

Ouellette H. The signet ring sign. Radiology 1999;212(1):67–68

Case 88

Brody AS, Klein JS, Molina PL, Quan J, Bean JA, Wilmott RW. High-resolution computed tomography in young patients with cystic fibrosis: distribution of abnormalities and correlation with pulmonary function tests. J Pediatr 2004;145(1):32–38

Ouellette H. The signet ring sign. Radiology 1999;212(1):67–68

Case 89

Miller BH, Rosado-de-Christenson ML, Mason AC, Fleming MV, White CC, Krasna MJ. From the archives of the AFIP. Malignant pleural mesothelioma: radiologic-pathologic correlation. Radiographics 1996;16(3):613–644

Roach HD, Davies GJ, Attanoos R, Crane M, Adams H, Phillips S. Asbestos: when the dust settles an imaging review of asbestos-related disease. Radiographics 2002;22(Spec No):S167–S184

Wang ZJ, Reddy GP, Gotway MB, et al. Malignant pleural mesothelioma: evaluation with CT, MR imaging, and PET. Radiographics 2004;24(1):105–119

Case 90

Koyama T, Ueda H, Togashi K, Umeoka S, Kataoka M, Nagai S. Radiologic manifestations of sarcoidosis in various organs. Radiographics 2004;24(1):87–104

Miller BH, Rosado-de-Christenson ML, McAdams HP, Fishback NF. Thoracic sarcoidosis: radiologic-pathologic correlation. Radiographics 1995;15(2):421–437

Prabhakar HB, Rabinowitz CB, Gibbons FK, O'Donnell WJ, Shepard JA, Aquino SL. Imaging features of sarcoidosis on MDCT, FDG PET, and PET/CT. AJR Am J Roentgenol 2008; 190(3, Suppl):S1–S6

Traill ZC, Maskell GF, Gleeson FV, High-Resolution CT. High-resolution CT findings of pulmonary sarcoidosis. AJR Am J Roentgenol 1997;168(6):1557–1560

Case 91

Kuhlman JE, Singha NK. Complex disease of the pleural space: radiographic and CT evaluation. Radiographics 1997;17(1):63–79

Roach HD, Davies GJ, Attanoos R, Crane M, Adams H, Phillips S. Asbestos: when the dust settles an imaging review of asbestos-related disease. Radiographics 2002;22(Spec No):S167–S184

Case 92

Hunter TB, Taljanovic MS, Tsau PH, Berger WG, Standen JR. Medical devices of the chest. Radiographics 2004;24(6):1725–1746

Shepherd MP. Plombage in the 1980s. Thorax 1985;40(5):328–340

Case 93

Engelke C, Schaefer-Prokop C, Schirg E, Freihorst J, Grubnic S, Prokop M. High-resolution CT and CT angiography of peripheral pulmonary vascular disorders. Radiographics 2002;22(4):739–764

Frazier AA, Galvin JR, Franks TJ, Rosado-De-Christenson ML. From the archives of the AFIP: pulmonary vasculature: hypertension and infarction. Radiographics 2000;20(2):491–524, quiz 530–531, 532

Case 94

Engelke C, Schaefer-Prokop C, Schirg E, Freihorst J, Grubnic S, Prokop M. High-resolution CT and CT angiography of peripheral pulmonary vascular disorders. Radiographics 2002;22(4):739–764

Frazier AA, Franks TJ, Mohammed TL, Ozbudak IH, Galvin JR. From the Archives of the AFIP: pulmonary veno-occlusive disease and pulmonary capillary hemangiomatosis. Radiographics 2007;27(3):867–882

Frazier AA, Galvin JR, Franks TJ, Rosado-De-Christenson ML. From the archives of the AFIP: pulmonary vasculature: hypertension and infarction. Radiographics 2000;20(2):491–524, quiz 530–531, 532

Case 95

Lee EY, Siegel MJ, Chu CM, Gutierrez FR, Kort HW. Amplatzer atrial septal defect occluder for pediatric patients: radiographic appearance. Radiology 2004;233(2):471–476

Wang ZJ, Reddy GP, Gotway MB, Yeh BM, Higgins CB. Cardiovascular shunts: MR imaging evaluation. Radiographics 2003;23(Spec No):S181–S194

Case 96

Frazier AA, Galvin JR, Franks TJ, Rosado-De-Christenson ML. From the archives of the AFIP: pulmonary vasculature: hypertension and infarction. Radiographics 2000;20(2):491–524, quiz 530–531, 532

Wang ZJ, Reddy GP, Gotway MB, Yeh BM, Higgins CB. Cardiovascular shunts: MR imaging evaluation. Radiographics 2003;23(Spec No):S181–S194

Case 97

Guttentag AR, Salwen JK. Keep your eyes on the ribs: the spectrum of normal variants and diseases that involve the ribs. Radiographics 1999;19(5):1125–1142

Kumar R, Madewell JE, Lindell MM, Swischuk LE. Fibrous lesions of bones. Radiographics 1990;10(2):237–256

Tateishi U, Gladish GW, Kusumoto M, et al. Chest wall tumors: radiologic findings and pathologic correlation: part 1. Benign tumors. Radiographics 2003;23(6):1477–1490

Case 98

Guttentag AR, Salwen JK. Keep your eyes on the ribs: the spectrum of normal variants and diseases that involve the ribs. Radiographics 1999;19(5):1125–1142

Tateishi U, Gladish GW, Kusumoto M, et al. Chest wall tumors: radiologic findings and pathologic correlation: part 2. Malignant tumors. Radiographics 2003;23(6):1491–1508

Case 99

Boiselle PM, Mansilla AV, Fisher MS, McLoud TC. Wandering wires: frequency of sternal wire abnormalities in patients with sternal dehiscence. AJR Am J Roentgenol 1999;173(3):777–780

Jolles H, Henry DA, Roberson JP, Cole TJ, Spratt JA. Mediastinitis following median sternotomy: CT findings. Radiology 1996;201(2):463–466

Case 100

Bruzzi JF, Komaki R, Walsh GL, et al. Imaging of non-small cell lung cancer of the superior sulcus: part 1: anatomy, clinical manifestations, and management. Radiographics 2008;28(2):551–560, quiz 620

Bruzzi JF, Komaki R, Walsh GL, et al. Imaging of non-small cell lung cancer of the superior sulcus: part 2: initial staging and assessment of resectability and therapeutic response. Radiographics 2008;28(2):561–572

Index

Note: Locators refer to case number. Locators in **boldface** indicate primary diagnosis.